双 极
TWO OPPOSITES

佟欣
XIN TONG

1

Main text: Xin Tong

Chinese translation: Xin Tong

Book design: Xin Tong

Copyright © 2014 XIN TONG

E-mail: drxintongtcm@gmail.com

Website: http://www.drxintong.com

ISBN: 978-0-9914556-2-1

目录
CONTENTS

前言 8

PREFACE 9

作者简介 12

ABOUT THE AUTHOR 15

鸣谢 16

ACKNOWLEDGMENTS 17

1. 双极 20

1. The Two Opposites 21

2. 双极理论 22

2. The Theory of Two Opposites 23

3. 双极表现 24

  3.1 阴阳理论的双极表现 24

3. The Manifestation of the Two Opposites 25

  3.1. The Manifestation of the Two Opposite Theory of Yin and Yang 25

  3.2 五行理论的双极表现 30

  3.2. The Manifestation of the Two Opposite Theory of Five Elements 31

  3.3 脏腑理论的双极表现： 32

3.3. **The Manifestation of the Two Opposite Theory of Zang Fu 33**

3.4 气血津液理论的双极表现 **58**

3.4. **The Manifestation of the Two Opposite Theory of Qi, Blood and Body Fluid** **59**

3.5 经络理论的双极表现 **62**

3.5. **The Manifestation of the Two Opposite Theory of Jing Luo(这里是和上文一致用 jing luo 好，还是用 meridian 好？) ... 63**

3.6 疾病的双极表现 **66**

3.6. **The Manifestation of the Two Opposite Theory of Diseases 67**

4. **双极治则** **70**

4.1 基本治则 **70**

4.1.1 理法 **70**

4

4. The Therapeutic Principles of the Two Opposites 71

    4.1. The Basic Therapeutic Principles 71

        4.1.1. Regulation...71

        4.1.2 化法...72

        4.1.3 养法...72

        4.1.2. Resolving..73

        4.1.3. Improvement 73

    4.2 联合治则 74

        4.2.1 日间治则 74

    4.2. The Associated Therapeutic Principles 75

        4.2.1. Daytime Therapeutic Principles 75

        4.2.2 夜间治则 76

        4.2.2. Nighttime Therapeutic Principles 77

        4.2.3 阴阳双极治则简述 80

        4.2.3. Brief Description of the Yin Yang Therapeutic Principles of the Two Opposites 81

        4.2.4 脏腑双极治则简述 82

        4.2.4. Brief Description of the Zang Fu Therapeutic Principles of the Two Opposites 83

        4.2.5 气血津液双极治则简述 100

        4.2.5. Brief Description of the Qi Blood and Body Fluid Therapeutic Principles of the Two Opposites 101

5. 理论推演 102

5. The Theoretical Deduction 103

6. 理论思维导图 106

6. The Mind Map indicating the Reasoning of the Theory 107

7. 病例举证 **112**

   7.1   病例 1 112

7.   Case Studies **113**

   7.1 Capse 1 113

   7.2   病例 2 ....**136**

   7.2 Case 2 ....**137**

   7.3   病例 3 ....**152**

   7.3 Case 3 ....**153**

   7.4   病例 4 ....**168**

   7.4 Case 4 ....**169**

参考文献 **182**

REFERENCES **183**

前言

我一直希望能够找到一些好的方法去学习和使用我所接触到的中医知识。但是由于中医体系过于庞大，如何学习和使用中医困扰了我多年。

PREFACE

I had been searching to find good ways to study Traditional Chinese Medicine and to use the knowledge I have acquired through experience in Traditional Chinese Medicine. Due to the enormous size of the theory of Traditional Chinese Medicine, the challenge of effectively learning and teaching Chinese medicine plagued me for years.

　　双极理论是在对我这十几年中医学习、使用所获得经验总结的基础上得来的。其灵感来自于"拆分"与"组合"两个词。"拆分"就是把那些看上去庞杂的体系打碎、拆开，然后按照最基本的规律去归类。"组合"就是把重新归类的碎片组合起来，还原原有体系或构建新体系的尝试。这个过程很有趣。因为这就好像搭积木，看上去我是在胡乱的堆砌，但在这个玩耍的过程中，我认识了每一块积木的特点。渐渐的从堆砌积木到搭建简单的模型，再到构建复杂体系。我在玩耍的过程中认识和掌握我所接触的一切。

The theory of Two Opposites is based on the culmination of my practical experience and years of study of Traditional Chinese Medicine. The inspiration comes from the two words "disassembly" and "combination". Disassembly is defined as, to breakdown a multifaceted disorderly system. I then follow basic rules and take that system apart to classify. "Combination" is defined as, to combine fragments or parts. These fragments are then combined, to restore the original system or try to build a new system. This process is very interesting, because it is like using building blocks. It may appear I am randomly combining blocks, but in the process of the play, I know the characteristics of each building block. Gradually I go from a pile of building blocks, to building a simple model, to building a complex system. I understand and master all my contact in the process of playing.

非常感谢您能阅读本书！如果您对本书有什么想法和建议，请给我发邮件。感谢您的关注！

佟欣

Thank you for your reading! If you have any ideas and suggestions about this book, please email me. Thank you for your attention!

Xin Tong

作者简介

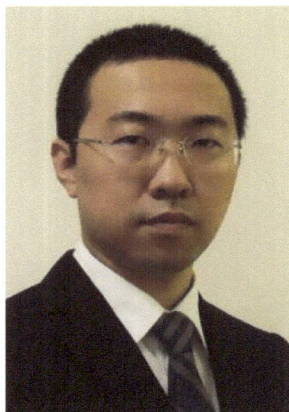

佟欣，毕业于黑龙江中医药大学，针灸推拿学硕士，中医执业医师。从事临床、教学和科研工作十余年。现任大西洋中医学院门诊主任、教授和针灸医师、世界中联儿科专业委员会第二届理事会理事、《走进新时代》特约编委和多家国际著名医学杂志审稿人。拥有针灸发明专利和多部中医专业著作，发表论文近三十篇。

ABOUT THE AUTHOR

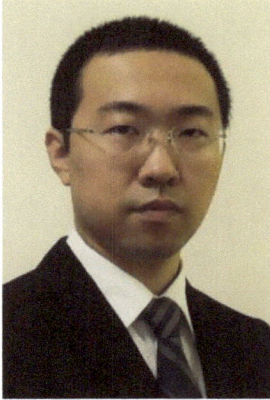

Dr. Xin Tong，Medical Doctor, Neurology (China), Acupuncture Physician, received his Chinese medicine education and his post-graduate training from Heilongjiang University of Traditional Chinese Medicine. He has engaged in clinical, teaching and scientific research work for more than ten years. At the present he holds the office of full time Acupuncture Physician, Clinic Director, Academic Professor at the Atlantic Institute of Oriental Medicine (ATOM), and Dr. Tong is a Council member of the New Council of 2nd board of directors of Pediatrics Specialty Committee (PSC) of World Federation of Chinese Medicine Societies (WFCMS), a contributing editor of "Towards a New Era" and reviewer of many famous international medical journals. Dr. Tong currently has a patent related to Acupuncture, a number of traditional Chinese medicine publications and more than 25 articles..

鸣谢

关于本书，我必须感谢我的母亲和父亲。在他们多年的鼓励和支持下，我从懵懂少年成长为一名医生。

另外还要致以我最诚挚的谢意于我的两位老师孙申田教授和孙忠人教授。是他们无私的将自己数十年的临床经验和教学经验传授给我；也是他们为我树立了为医和为师的典范；更是他们鼓励我来到大洋彼岸美国投身西方中医发展的工作中。

特别感谢大西洋中医学院朱海纳校长和付迪副校长在我写作本书期间给予的各方面支持。

ACKNOWLEDGMENTS

About this book, I would like to thank my mother and father for their encouragement and support all these years. For that, I grew up from a young boy to be a Doctor.

In addition I am grateful for two of my teachers. One is Professor Shentian Sun, the other is Professor Zhongren Sun. Both of them are prominent scholars at the Heilongjiang University of Traditional Chinese Medicine. They were selfless to teach me their decades of clinical experience and teaching experience. They are the model of doctor and teacher in my mind. Furthermore, they encouraged me to travel across the ocean to assist in the future development of Chinese Medicine in the West.

Special gratitude should go to Dr. Johanna Yen, President of the Atlantic Institute of Oriental Medicine, and Dr. Fu Di, Vice President of the Institute for their help in all aspects of support.

感谢陈鑫柏教授和我的学生温迪.米勒、玛丽亚.劳拉.雷纳在全书翻译过程中给予的大量帮助。

最后要感谢我的挚爱、我的夫人刘丹丹女士。这本书的诞生完全来自于她的鼓励。是她在我对过去经验总结的过程中清晰地捕捉到了双极理论的特点，使我明确了研究方向，总结、整理、构建和完善了双极理论体系；也是她在精神和生活上给予我最大的支持，使我能够完成本书。

Special mention must be made of the help rendered by Professor Xinbo Chen，my students Wendy Miller and Maria Laura Rainer who gives assistance in the translation process of the book.

Finally I want to thank my love, my wife Dandan Liu. The birth of the book completely came from her encouragement. She clearly captured the characteristics of the theory of two opposites when I was summing up the experiences of the past. That made me found the research direction, and summarized, systemized, built and perfected the theory of two opposite system. Therefore, with her great support of spirit and life, I could finish this book.

1. 双极

顾名思义，两个极端。在双极理论中双极代表的是世间万物和人体的阴阳。在中医理论上，双极的现实表现为日夜中不同的症状、治则和治疗方法。而其理论表现为阴阳之间的各种关系，并以此为基础演化为阴阳双极理论、脏腑双极理论、气血津液双极理论、经络双极理论，疾病双极理论，五行理论由于源于阴阳理论，并融入于脏腑理论中，故不单独区分五行双极理论。

1. The Two Opposites

"Shuang Ji(双极)" stands for the two extremes or rather, the two opposites in philosophy. The opposites are represented by Yin and Yang, which can be used to categorize all things in the world, including the human body. According to Traditional Chinese Medicine (TCM) Theory, the realistic expression of the Opposites Theory means that symptoms, therapeutic principles and treatments differ between day and night. The theoretic expression means all the relationships are between Yin and Yang. The Opposites Theory generates Yin Yang, Zang Fu, Qi Blood and Body Fluid, Jing Luo and Disease Opposites theories. Note that the Five Element Theory is derived directly from the Yin Yang theory and is combined with the Zang Fu theory, it is therefore not listed separately.

2. 双极理论

　　理论和现实的双极表现结合在一起为双极理论的理论基础；日夜分治的双极治则为双极理论的实践基础。理论基础揭示了阴阳、脏腑、气血津液、经络和疾病的日夜运行规律。实践基础则对日夜分治的治则和治法做出解释。将以上两个基础相结合，形成理论指导实践，实践反作用于理论的相辅相成的理论。我将它命名为"双极理论"。

2. The Theory of Two Opposites

The theoretical basis of the Two Opposites is the combination of the theoretical expression and realistic expression. The practical basis of the Two Opposites Theory is its therapeutic principles, which divide the therapeutic principles adopted for the daytime from the therapeutic principles applicable for night.   The theoretical basis is used to explain the variable working process of Yin Yang, Zang Fu, Qi Blood and Body Fluid, Jing Luo and Disease in the day and night. The practical basis explains the variations of therapeutic principles and treatments in the day and night. The combination of these two leads to the formation of the theory in which the theory gives guidance to practices, but at the same time, practices can also affect theory. Thus, I call this a "Theory of the Two Opposites".

3. 双极表现

3.1 阴阳理论的双极表现

中医的核心理论为阴阳理论，它是论述其他一切理论的基础。正如《素问·阴阳应象大论》所说的"阴阳者，天地之道也，万物之纲纪，变化之父母，生杀之本始，神明之府也，治病必求之本"。因此，阴阳理论是双极理论的核心思想。

3. The Manifestation of the Two Opposites

3.1. The Manifestation of the Two Opposite Theory of Yin and Yang

Yin and Yang theory is the core of Traditional Chinese Medical (TCM). It is the fundamental theoretical basis for the explanation of all other TCM theories. Just as *Su Wen - Great Topic on Correspondences and Manifestation of Yin and Yang writes:* *"The Principle of Yin and yang is the universal truth of the world, the essence of everything under the Sun. It is the mother of all changes as well as the beginning and ending of life and death and it is the palace of our mind and spirit. Therefore, when it comes to the treatment of illnesses, we must strive to get at the core of them."* Hence, the theory of Yin and Yang is the core of the Two – Opposite Theory.

阴阳理论的"双极表现"表现为昼夜间人体阴阳之间的转化规律。黎明时分随着太阳的升起，人体的阳气逐渐旺盛，温煦和推动全身血液和津液的运行加速，促使脏腑和经络由夜间的静默修养状态转换为日间的积极工作状态。在正午时分阳气的旺盛状态达到巅峰。午后阳气由盛转衰，随太阳的西垂而逐渐转入收藏状态。至夜半三更，人体的阳气完全内敛于内，为次日的再次升腾蓄积能量。

The manifestation of Yin and Yang theory clearly indicates the transformation rule of elements inside the human body between daytime and night time. As the sun rises at dawn, human body's Yang also increases accordingly. It warms up, promotes and speeds up blood circulation as well as the body fluid circulation from head to toe. Meanwhile, it would change the still, quiet status of the Zang-Fu organs and meridian system into the active working status. At noon time, Yang rises and increases to its peak. However, in the afternoon, following the setting sun, Yang would start to decline changing from the flourish status into the status of storage. It will continue it's transformation to the status of complete hiding and storage inside the human body at midnight. During this process, Yang accumulates energy for tomorrow's rebirth or re-rising.

　　阴血同样追随阳气的日夜变化而变化。不同的是在整个过程中，日间阴血追随阳气的变化而变化；而夜间阴血则濡润阳气，助阳气收藏。阴阳这种夜伏昼出迥然相异的极端转化规律，正是双极理论中"双极表现"的核心表现。同时与《素问·阴阳应象大论》所说的"阳生阴长，阳杀阴藏"相吻合。

Yin has almost the same circulation as Yang. However, there are some differences. Yin's movement follows Yang's movement in the daytime. Yin tonifies Yang, helping it to hide and maintain the status of quietness and storage through-out the entire night. This difference of extreme transformation rule of Yin and Yang between the daytime, being very active and the night being hidden is the core manifestation of the performance in the Two-Opposite Theory. This is supported and confirmed with evidence in *Su Wen: "Yin grows while Yang generates, Yin concedes when Yang is restrained".*

3.2五行理论的双极表现

五行以阴阳转化为基础，表现于脏腑、气血津液和经络理论中，故不做单独讨论。

3.2. The Manifestation of the Two Opposite Theory of Five Elements

Five elements are based on Yin and Yang transformation and transportation and fully reflected in Zang Fu theory, Qi Blood and Essential Body Fluid theory and Jing Luo theory. Therefore, it will not be discussed as a separate section.

3.3脏腑理论的双极表现：

　　脏、腑和奇恒之府，由于受到阴阳的直接影响，其功能虽然各不相同，但是总体上依然遵循夜伏昼出的规律。但是仍需指出的是，以下几个脏腑并非夜间完全处于封藏或静默状态。它们是心、肾、脑、髓。

3.3. The Manifestation of the Two Opposite Theory of Zang Fu

Zang-Fu and Extraordinary organs are influenced directly by Yin and Yang. Their functions are different from each other, but in general they still follow the same rule of Yin and Yang. During the daytime they are very active and become hidden in the night. Nevertheless, it is necessary to point out that the following organs are not completely in the hidden status at night. They are the heart, kidney, brain and marrow. These organs continue to function in a more active state.

心，主神志。而脑对于神志的影响也非常巨大。二者在夜间依然对神志的运行发挥着作用。只不过，这种作用有别于日间的统摄，而更趋向于梳理和引导。在这个过程中，心和脑将日间和过去所经历的各种正面的和负面的思绪进行分类，并将有用的部分转化为记忆储存起来，而无用的部分则选择被忘记。它们工作的这一过程表现在现实生活中，就是梦境。

While the heart dominates spirit, the brain also has great influence on spirit during the daytime. Both the heart and brain will continue to work at night in a different capacity. They tend to focus on regulating and guiding spirit at night. In this process, heart and brain first classify the positive and negative thinking of the daytime or past. In addition, they will transform the useful parts of thinking and store them in the memory. For things they deem useless, they will choose to forget about them and not store these things. In the realistic life, the whole working process of heart and brain is manifested in our dreams.

　　肾脏由于是人体阴阳的根本，它肩负着统摄人体阴阳平衡的重任。所以即使在夜间，肾脏也不可能停止工作。只不过是工作的重点从日间协调阴阳在人体各部的分配转移到促进阴阳之间的转化，加强阴阳在夜间的封藏以及对其它各个脏腑在夜间休养生息的管理。

As kidney is the root of the human body's Yin and Yang, its important task is to dominate and balance Yin and Yang. So even at night, kidney will never stop working. The difference is that the focus of the work is now shifted from coordinating the distribution of Yin and Yang to improving the inter-transformation of Yin and Yang into the various parts of the body. The kidney works to reinforce the energy collection and storage of Yin and Yang, as well as reinforcing the supervision of the handling of the rest and revitalization of other organs at night.

　　髓包含脑，但是脑是髓中比较特别的部分。因为脑和心一起作用，统摄神志。但是总体来说脑和髓本质是相同的，它们接受肾中精气滋养，然后滋养骨骼和神志。而这个滋养的过程主要发生在夜间。日间除脑以外的髓的活动相对减少，只在特殊情况下，如意外大量失血，失津的情况下，才会活动加剧。所以髓的功能是有别于其它脏腑的。但其日夜功能状态的迥然不同依然符合双极理论的"双极表现"。

　　下面将脏腑理论的双极表现简述如下：

Brain is a special part of marrow. It works with heart in dominating spirit. The main functionality of the brain and marrow are essentially the same. They are nourished by kidney essence and in turn they nourish bones and spirit. This nourishing process usually occurs at night. The activities of marrow will relatively slow down in the daytime except the functions of the brain. Only in special cases, such as accidental massive blood and body fluid loss, will the activities of marrow increase. Therefore, the function of marrow is different from the functions of other organs. This extremely different functional status of marrow is also in accordance with the manifestation of the Two-Opposite Theory.

The manifestation of the two - opposite theory of Zang Fu is basically as follows:

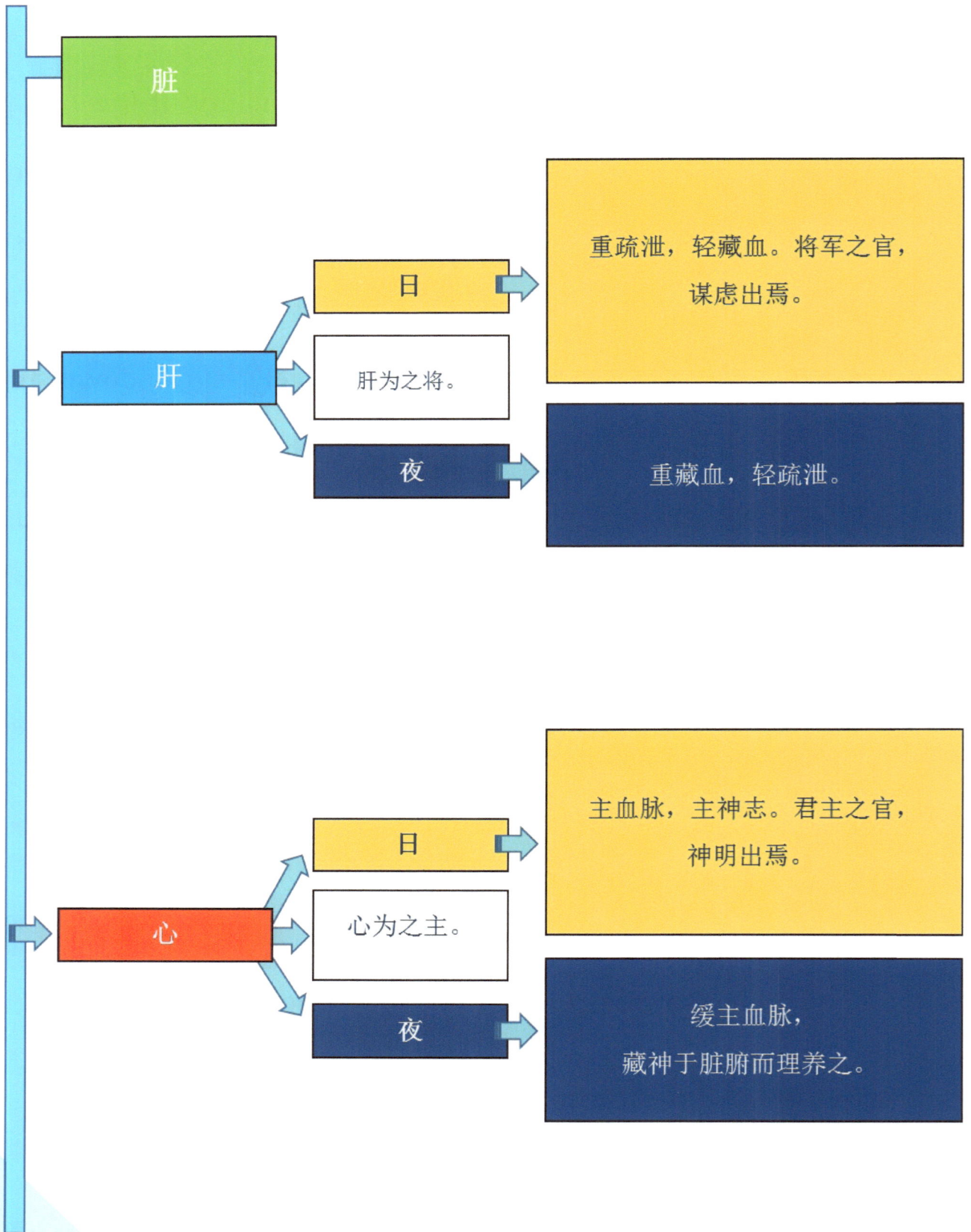

脏

肝

日 → 重疏泄，轻藏血。将军之官，谋虑出焉。

肝为之将。

夜 → 重藏血，轻疏泄。

心

日 → 主血脉，主神志。君主之官，神明出焉。

心为之主。

夜 → 缓主血脉，藏神于脏腑而理养之。

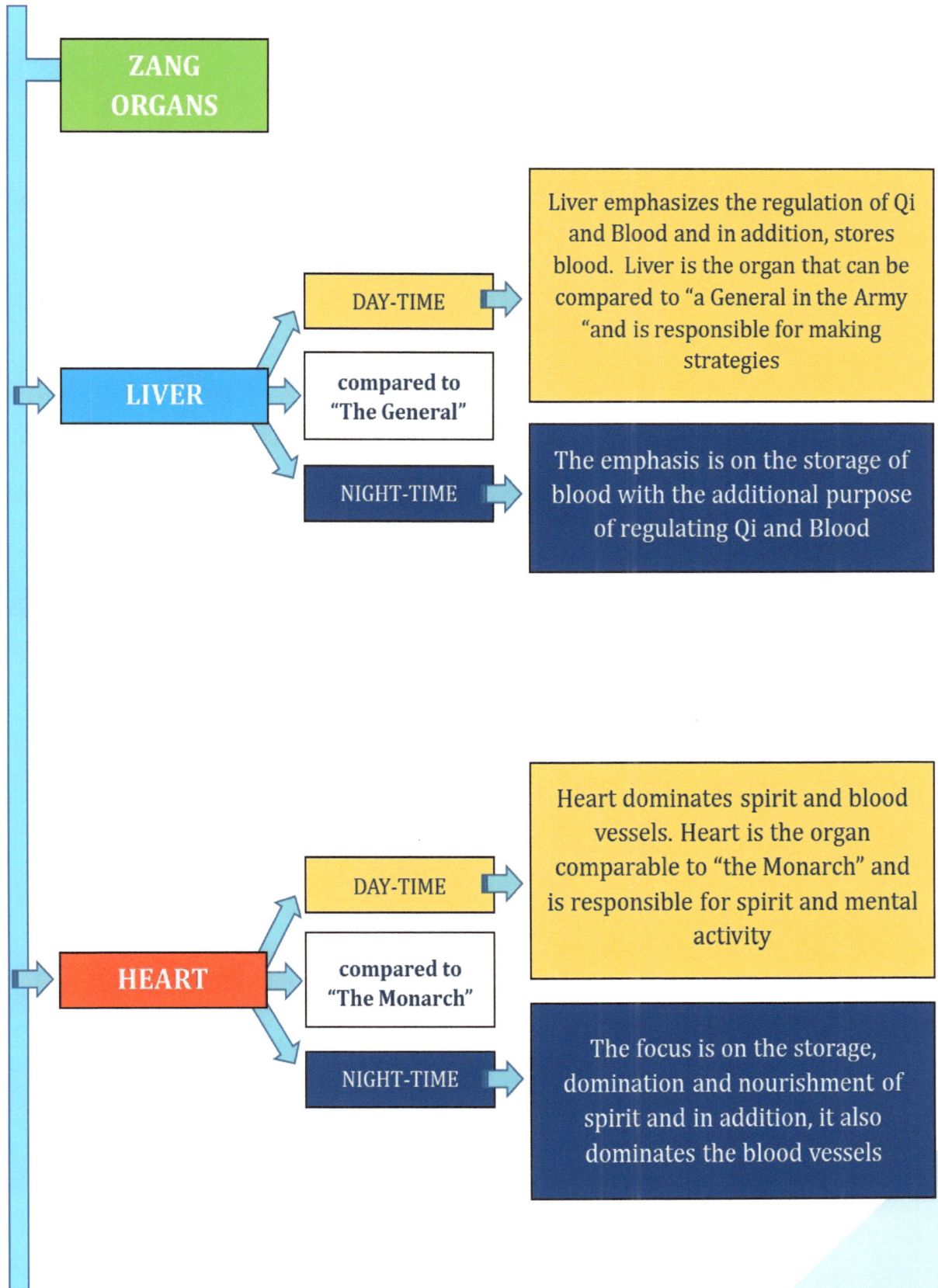

ZANG ORGANS

LIVER

DAY-TIME → Liver emphasizes the regulation of Qi and Blood and in addition, stores blood. Liver is the organ that can be compared to "a General in the Army "and is responsible for making strategies

compared to "The General"

NIGHT-TIME → The emphasis is on the storage of blood with the additional purpose of regulating Qi and Blood

HEART

DAY-TIME → Heart dominates spirit and blood vessels. Heart is the organ comparable to "the Monarch" and is responsible for spirit and mental activity

compared to "The Monarch"

NIGHT-TIME → The focus is on the storage, domination and nourishment of spirit and in addition, it also dominates the blood vessels

41

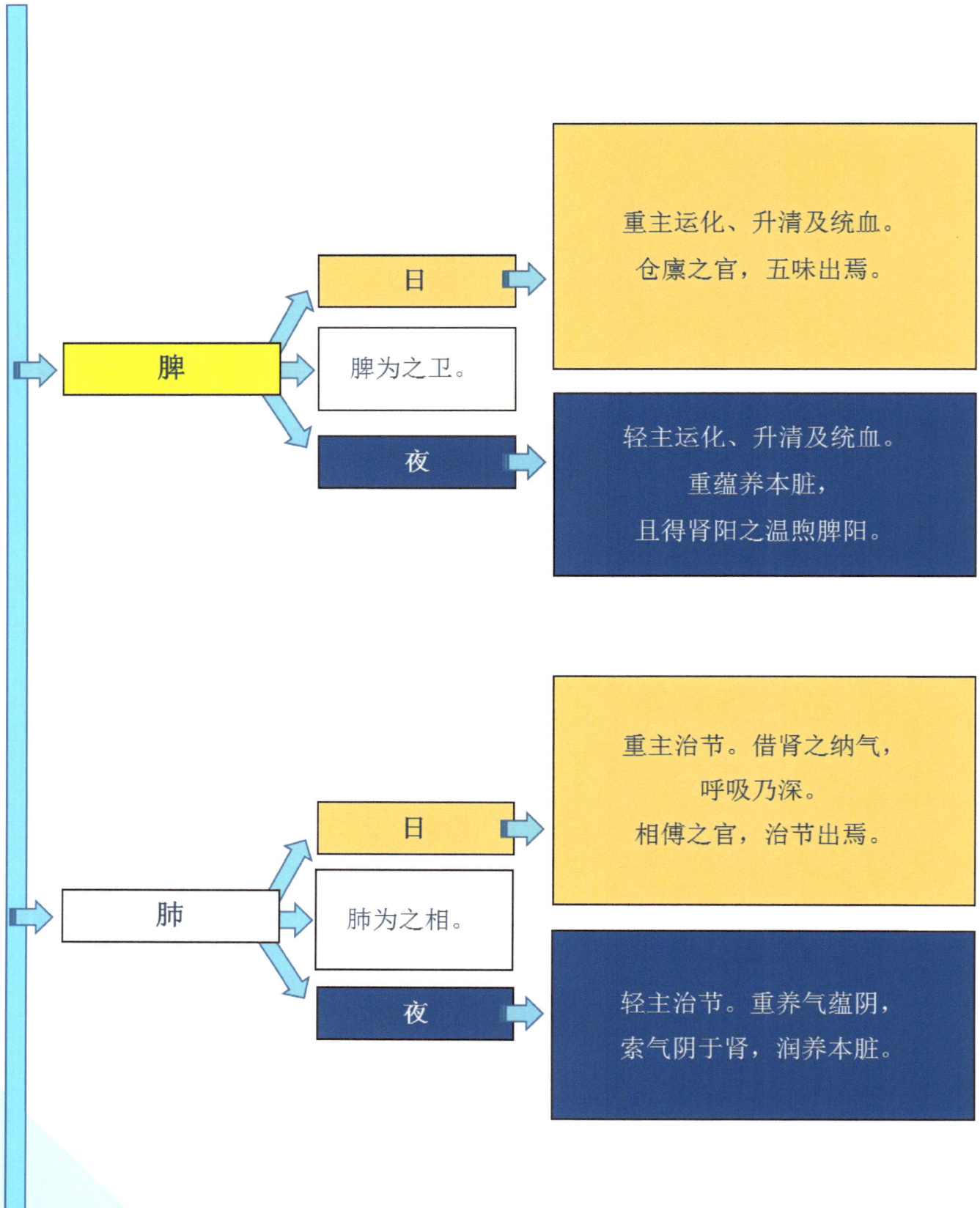

脾

日 → 重主运化、升清及统血。
仓廪之官，五味出焉。

脾为之卫。

夜 → 轻主运化、升清及统血。
重蕴养本脏，
且得肾阳之温煦脾阳。

肺

日 → 重主治节。借肾之纳气，
呼吸乃深。
相傅之官，治节出焉。

肺为之相。

夜 → 轻主治节。重养气蕴阴，
索气阴于肾，润养本脏。

42

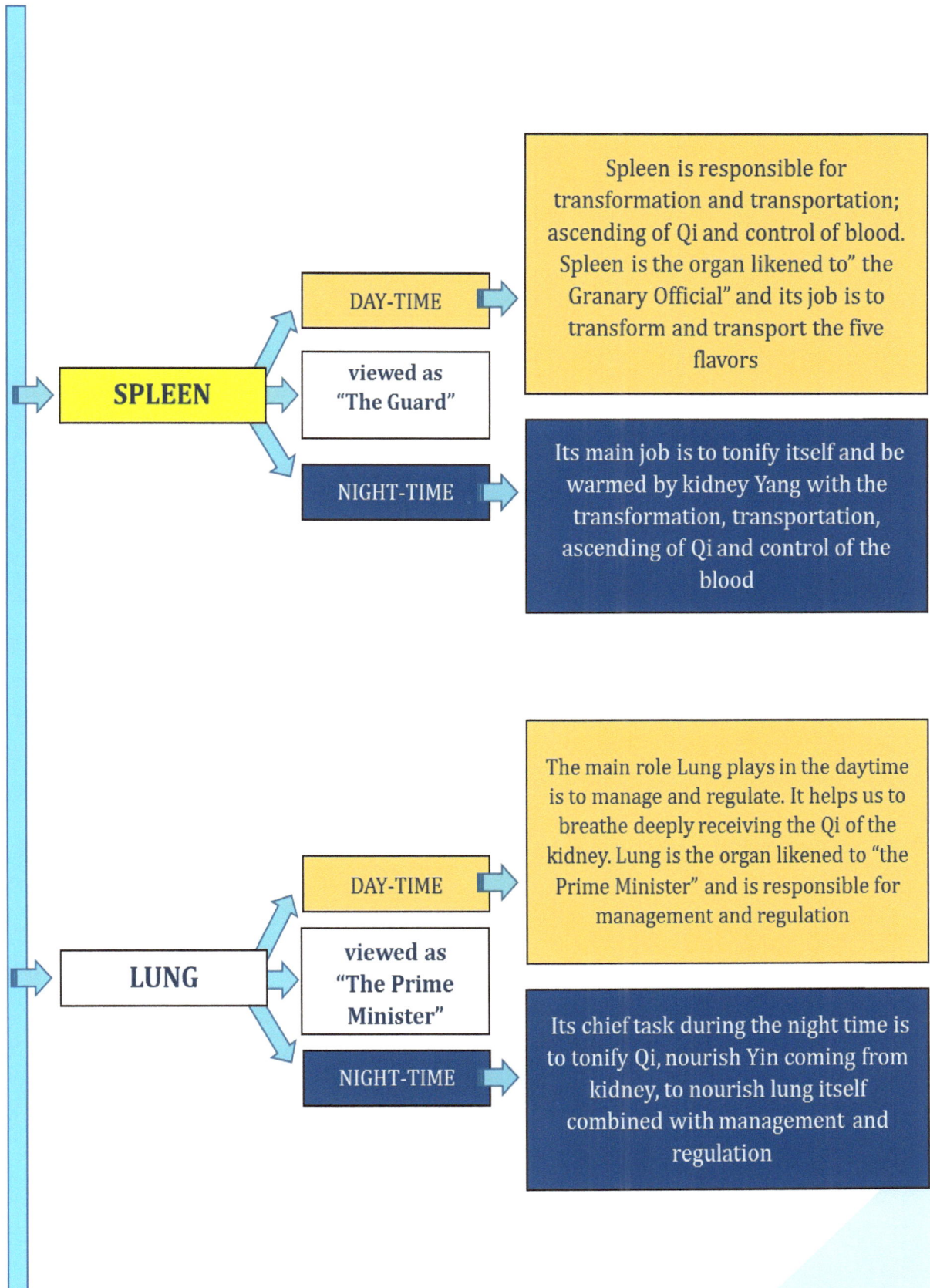

SPLEEN

viewed as "The Guard"

DAY-TIME → Spleen is responsible for transformation and transportation; ascending of Qi and control of blood. Spleen is the organ likened to" the Granary Official" and its job is to transform and transport the five flavors

NIGHT-TIME → Its main job is to tonify itself and be warmed by kidney Yang with the transformation, transportation, ascending of Qi and control of the blood

LUNG

viewed as "The Prime Minister"

DAY-TIME → The main role Lung plays in the daytime is to manage and regulate. It helps us to breathe deeply receiving the Qi of the kidney. Lung is the organ likened to "the Prime Minister" and is responsible for management and regulation

NIGHT-TIME → Its chief task during the night time is to tonify Qi, nourish Yin coming from kidney, to nourish lung itself combined with management and regulation

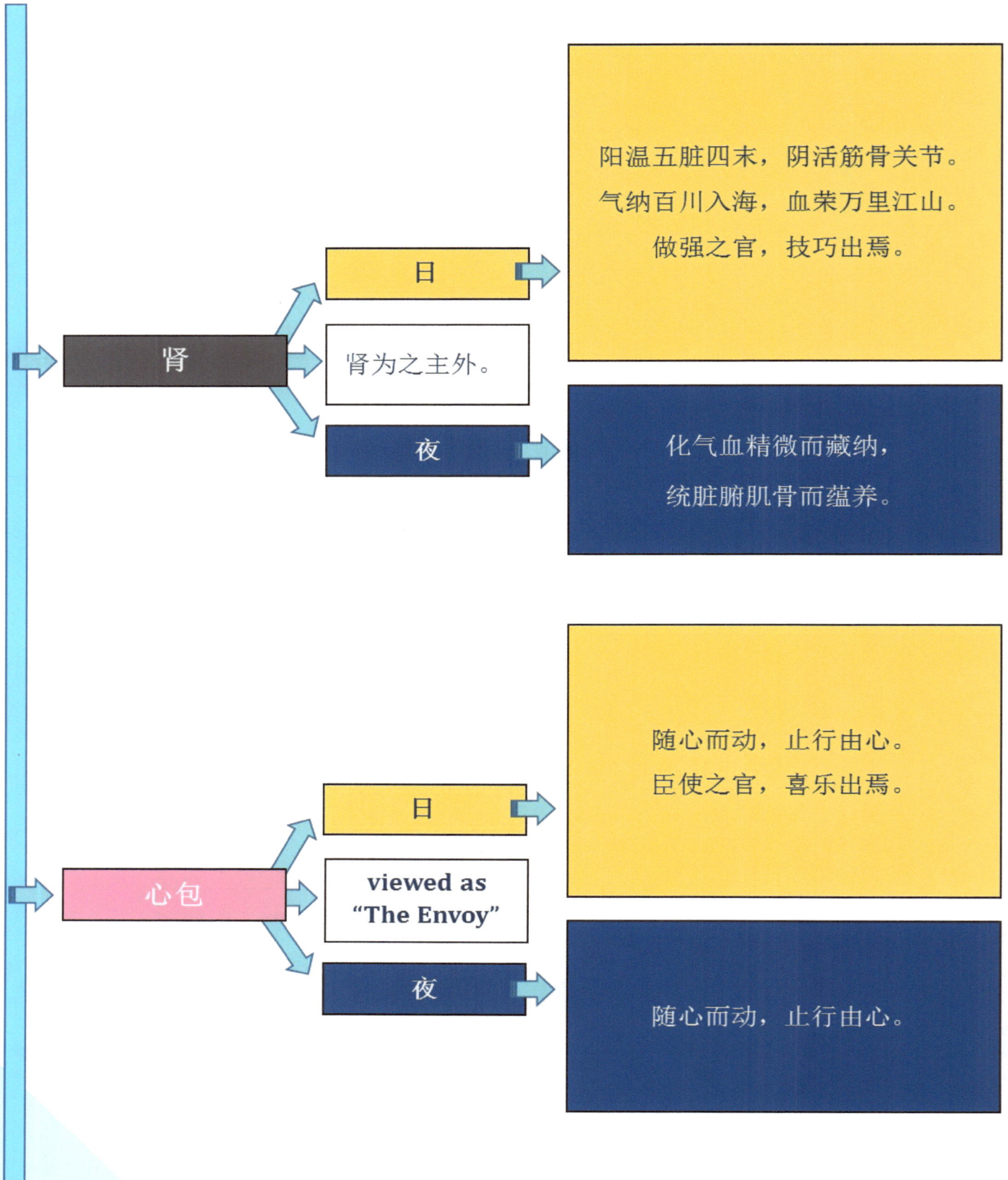

肾

日 → 阳温五脏四末，阴活筋骨关节。
气纳百川入海，血荣万里江山。
做强之官，技巧出焉。

肾为之主外。

夜 → 化气血精微而藏纳，
统脏腑肌骨而蕴养。

心包

日 → 随心而动，止行由心。
臣使之官，喜乐出焉。

viewed as
"The Envoy"

夜 → 随心而动，止行由心。

44

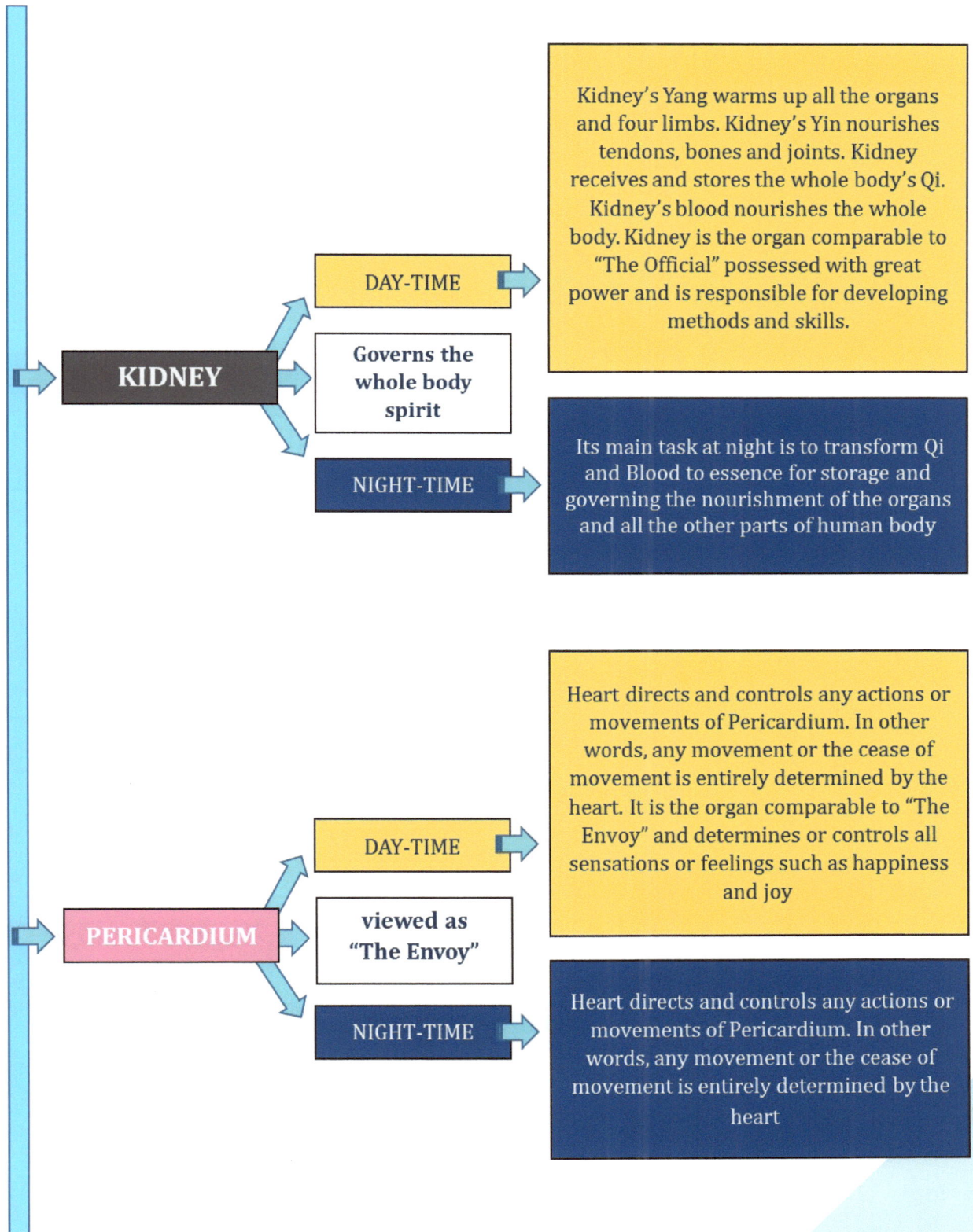

KIDNEY

DAY-TIME

Governs the whole body spirit

NIGHT-TIME

Kidney's Yang warms up all the organs and four limbs. Kidney's Yin nourishes tendons, bones and joints. Kidney receives and stores the whole body's Qi. Kidney's blood nourishes the whole body. Kidney is the organ comparable to "The Official" possessed with great power and is responsible for developing methods and skills.

Its main task at night is to transform Qi and Blood to essence for storage and governing the nourishment of the organs and all the other parts of human body

PERICARDIUM

DAY-TIME

viewed as "The Envoy"

NIGHT-TIME

Heart directs and controls any actions or movements of Pericardium. In other words, any movement or the cease of movement is entirely determined by the heart. It is the organ comparable to "The Envoy" and determines or controls all sensations or feelings such as happiness and joy

Heart directs and controls any actions or movements of Pericardium. In other words, any movement or the cease of movement is entirely determined by the heart

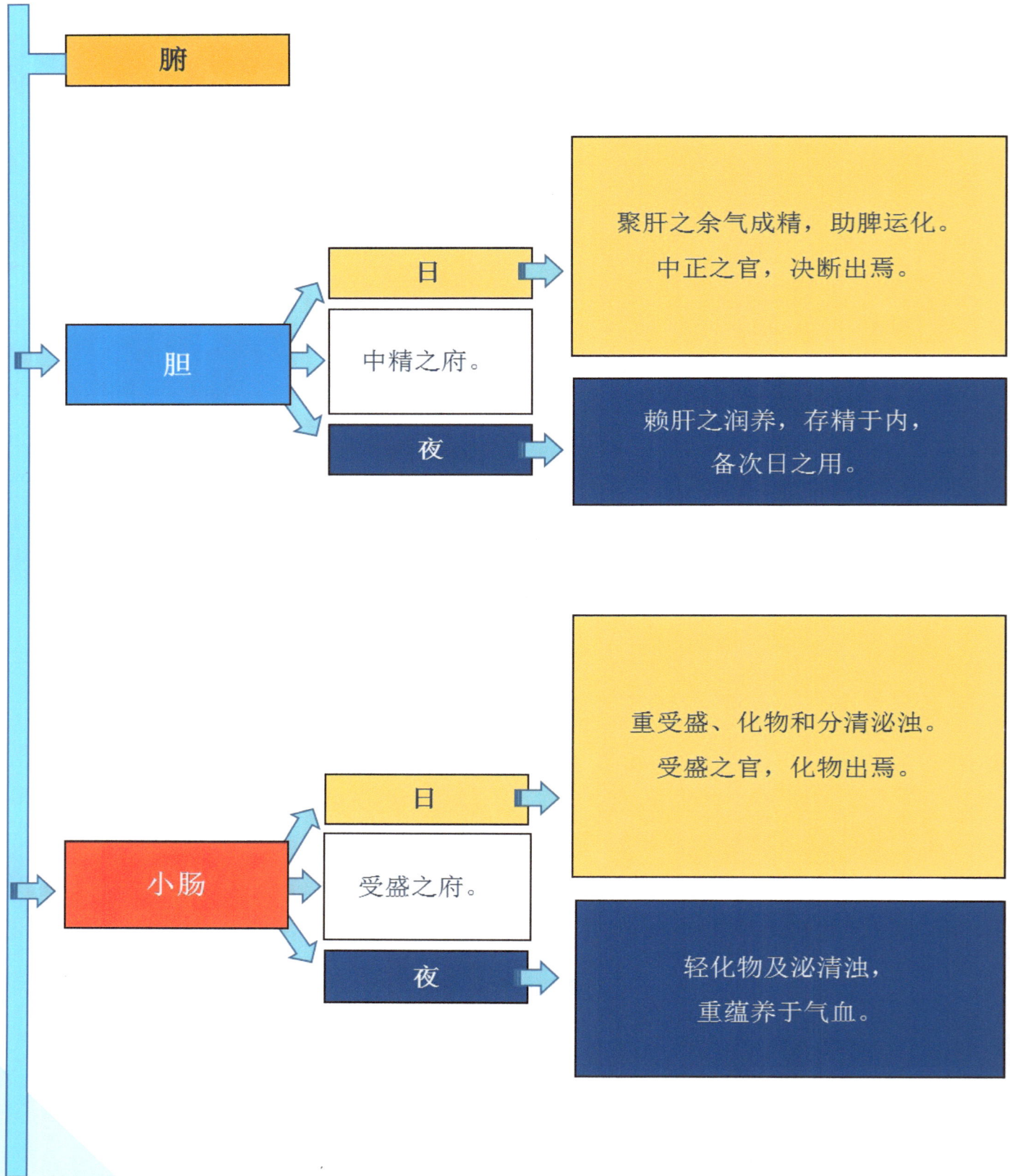

腑

胆

日 → 聚肝之余气成精，助脾运化。
中正之官，决断出焉。

中精之府。

夜 → 赖肝之润养，存精于内，
备次日之用。

小肠

日 → 重受盛、化物和分清泌浊。
受盛之官，化物出焉。

受盛之府。

夜 → 轻化物及泌清浊，
重蕴养于气血。

46

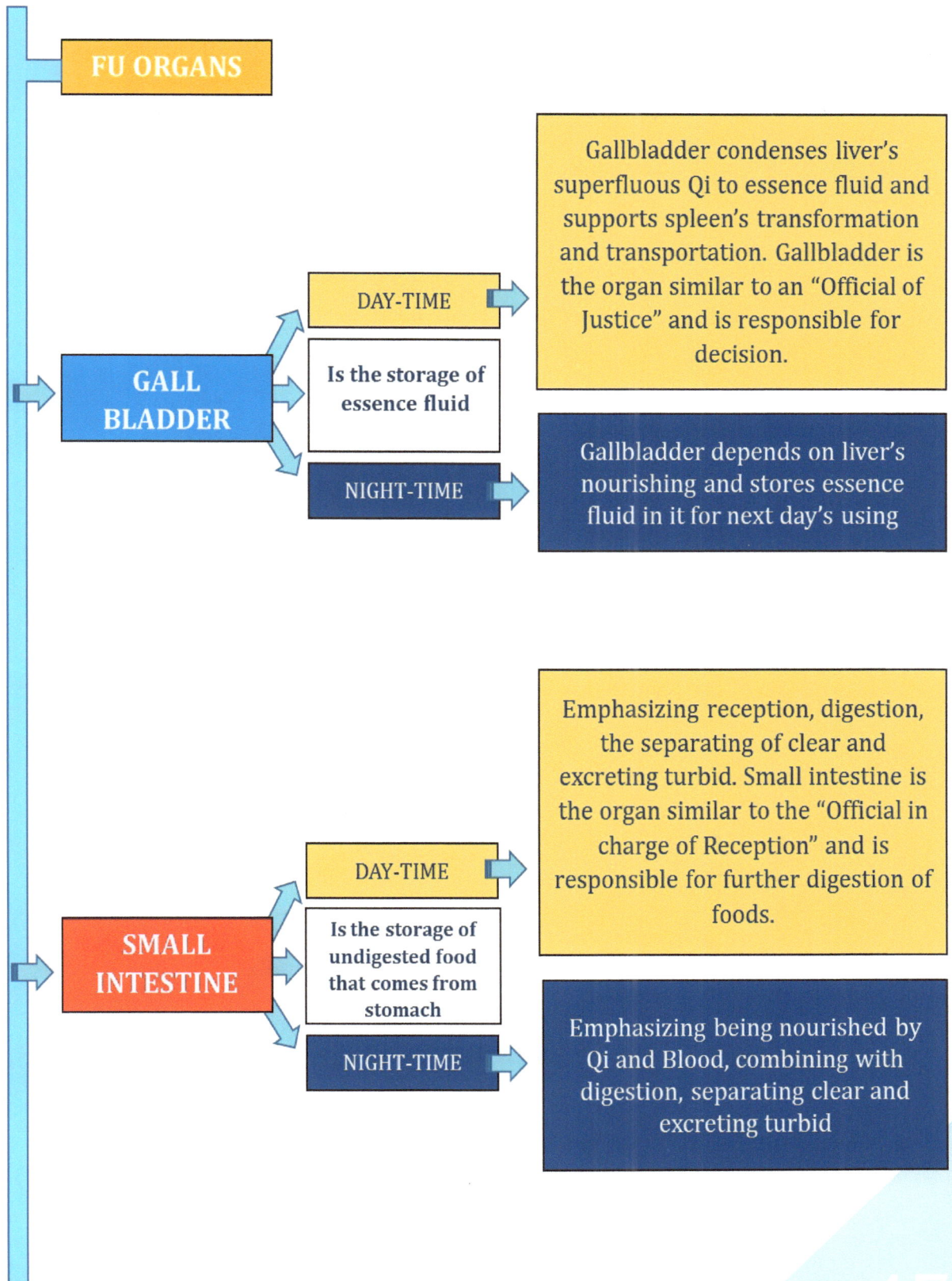

FU ORGANS

GALL BLADDER

DAY-TIME

Is the storage of essence fluid

NIGHT-TIME

Gallbladder condenses liver's superfluous Qi to essence fluid and supports spleen's transformation and transportation. Gallbladder is the organ similar to an "Official of Justice" and is responsible for decision.

Gallbladder depends on liver's nourishing and stores essence fluid in it for next day's using

SMALL INTESTINE

DAY-TIME

Is the storage of undigested food that comes from stomach

NIGHT-TIME

Emphasizing reception, digestion, the separating of clear and excreting turbid. Small intestine is the organ similar to the "Official in charge of Reception" and is responsible for further digestion of foods.

Emphasizing being nourished by Qi and Blood, combining with digestion, separating clear and excreting turbid

47

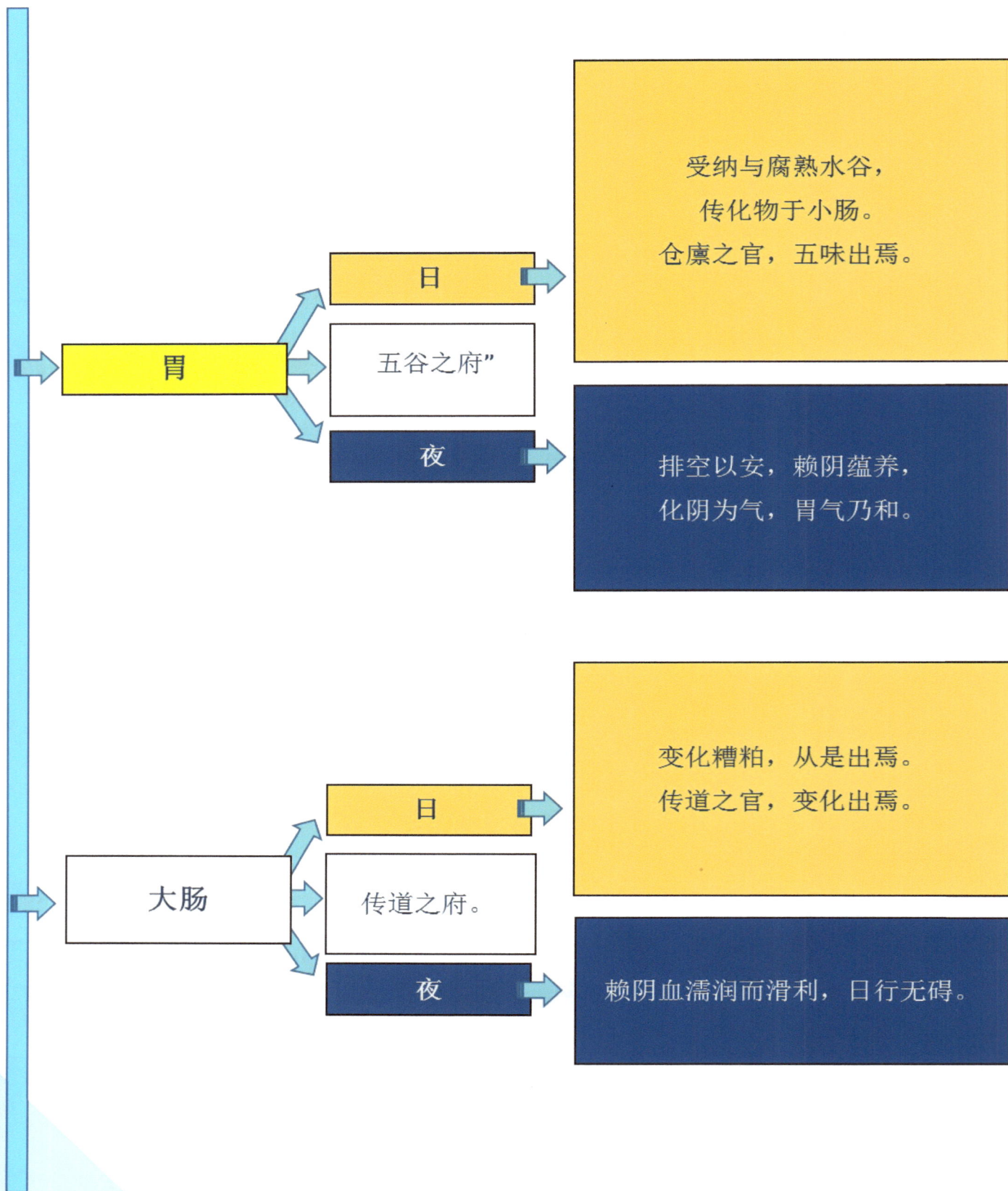

胃

日

五谷之府"

夜

受纳与腐熟水谷，
传化物于小肠。
仓廪之官，五味出焉。

排空以安，赖阴蕴养，
化阴为气，胃气乃和。

大肠

日

传道之府。

夜

变化糟粕，从是出焉。
传道之官，变化出焉。

赖阴血濡润而滑利，日行无碍。

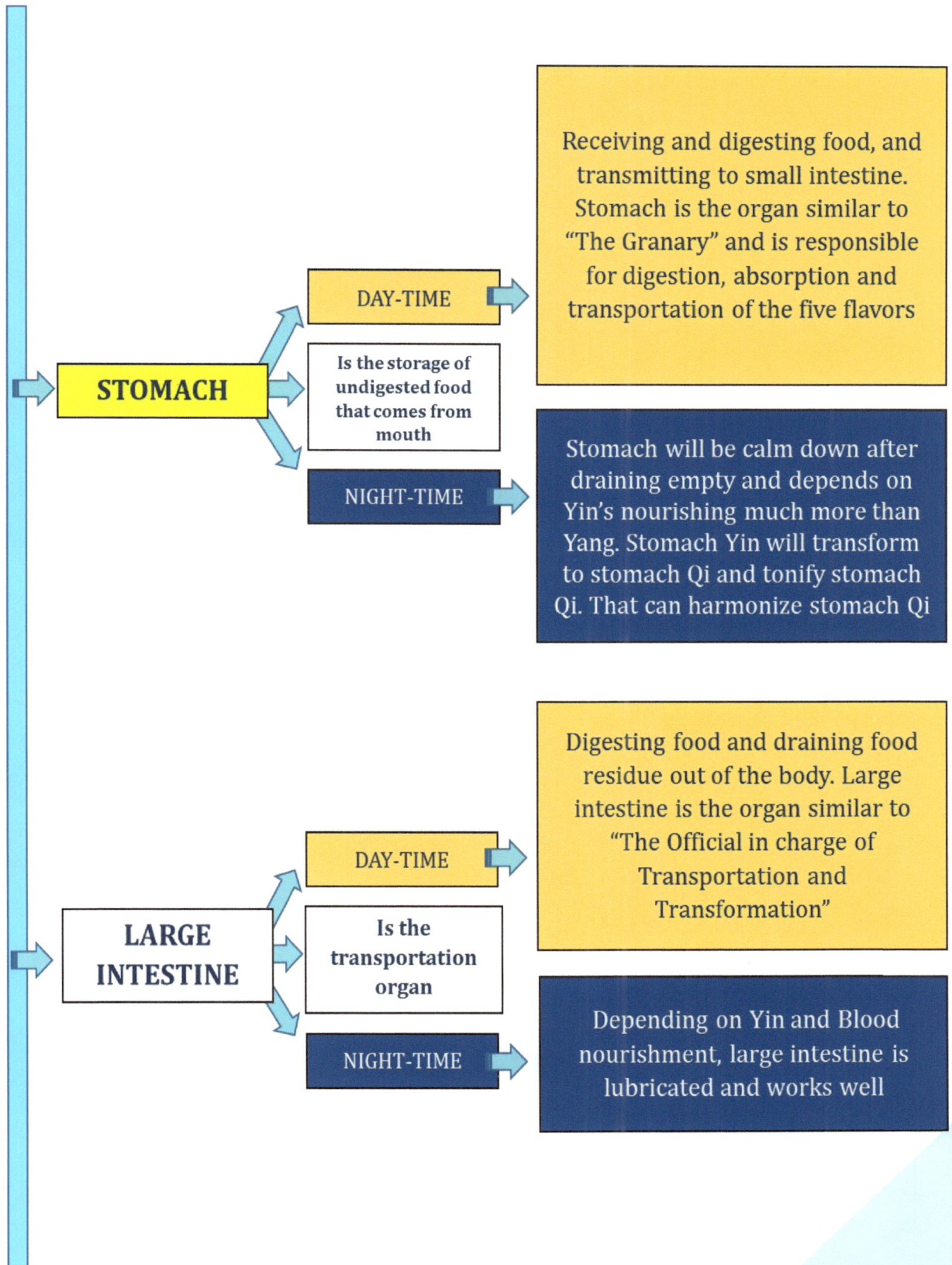

STOMACH

DAY-TIME → Receiving and digesting food, and transmitting to small intestine. Stomach is the organ similar to "The Granary" and is responsible for digestion, absorption and transportation of the five flavors

Is the storage of undigested food that comes from mouth

NIGHT-TIME → Stomach will be calm down after draining empty and depends on Yin's nourishing much more than Yang. Stomach Yin will transform to stomach Qi and tonify stomach Qi. That can harmonize stomach Qi

LARGE INTESTINE

DAY-TIME → Digesting food and draining food residue out of the body. Large intestine is the organ similar to "The Official in charge of Transportation and Transformation"

Is the transportation organ

NIGHT-TIME → Depending on Yin and Blood nourishment, large intestine is lubricated and works well

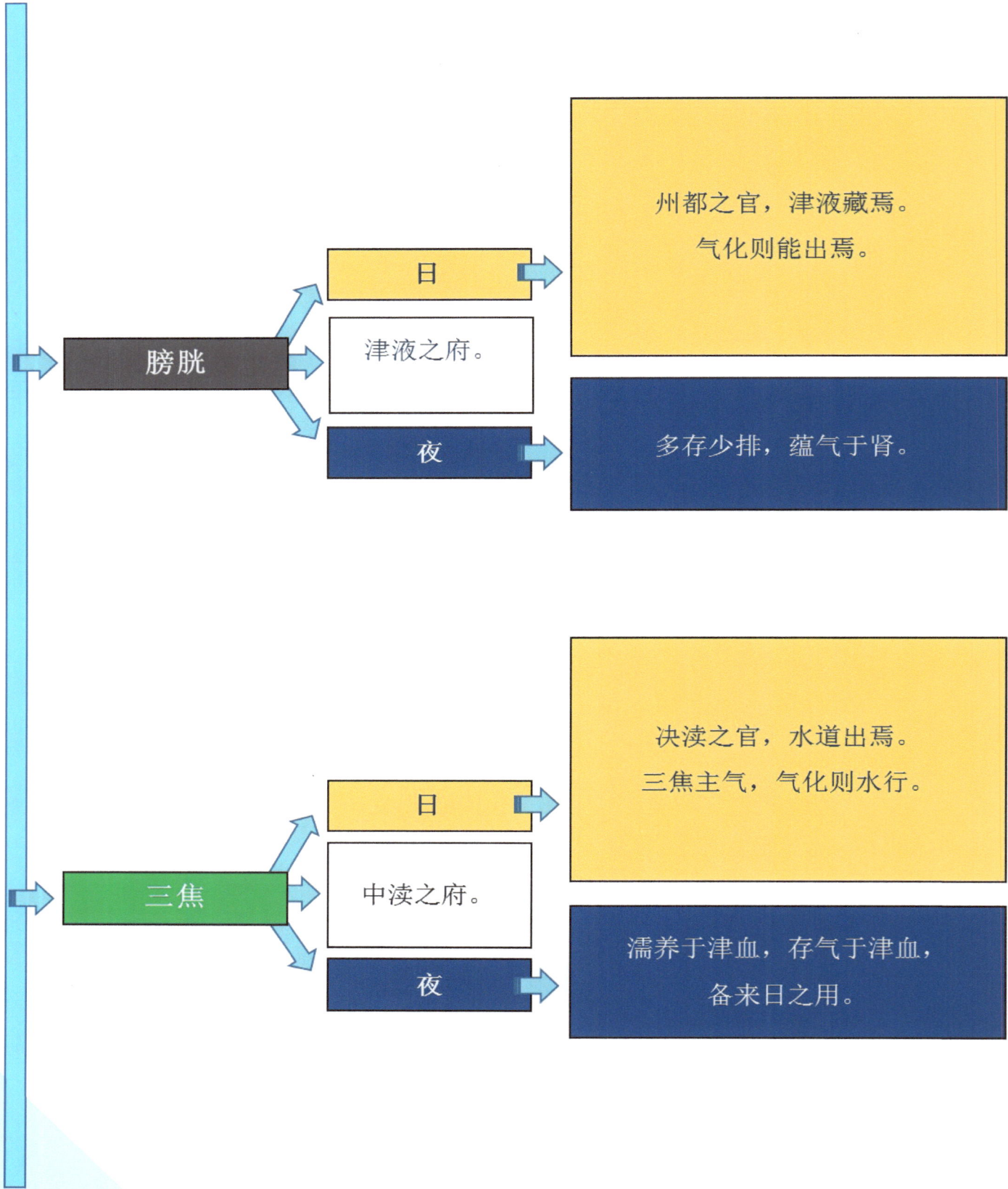

膀胱

日 → 州都之官，津液藏焉。
气化则能出焉。

津液之府。

夜 → 多存少排，蕴气于肾。

三焦

日 → 决渎之官，水道出焉。
三焦主气，气化则水行。

中渎之府。

夜 → 濡养于津血，存气于津血，
备来日之用。

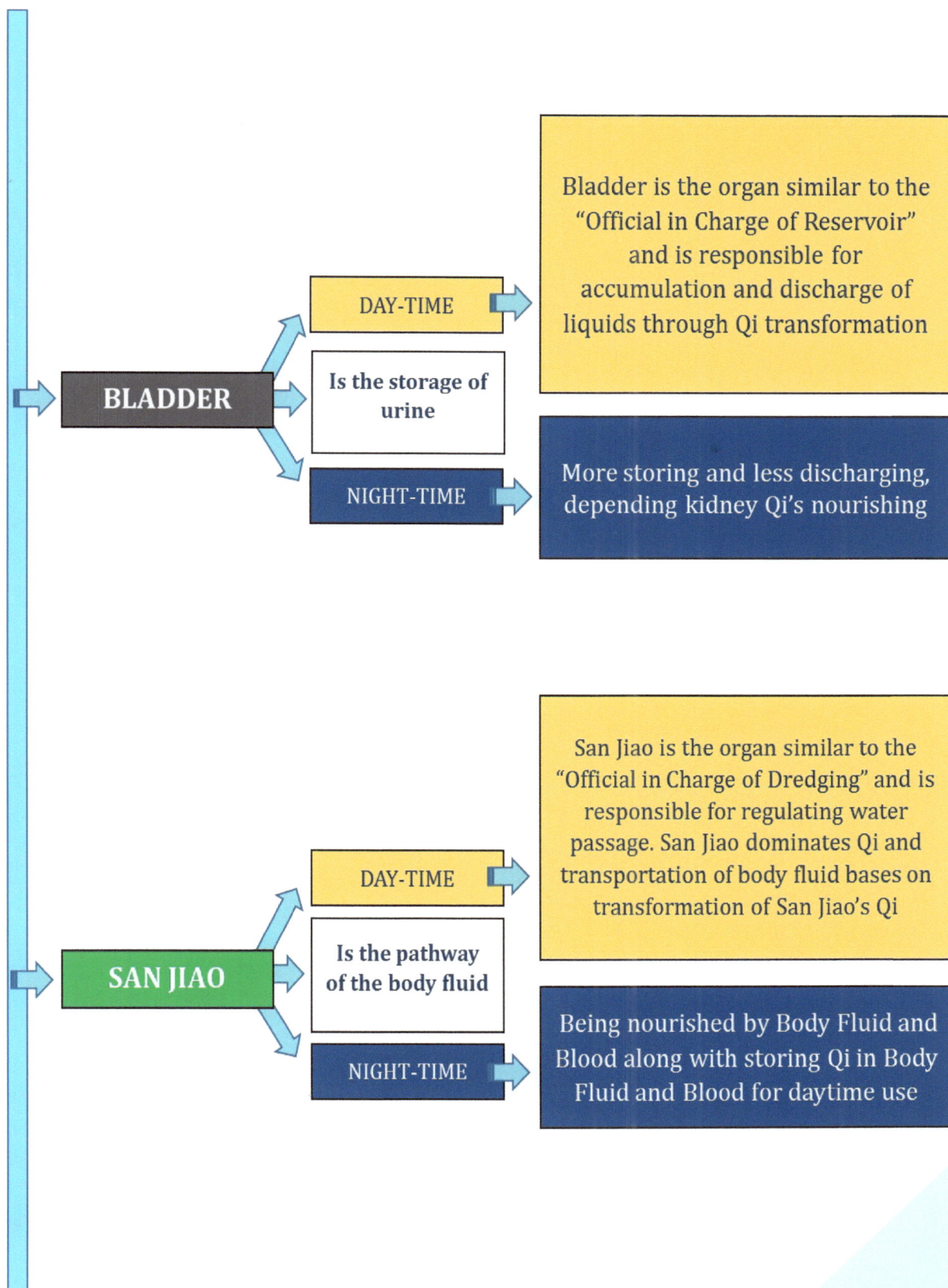

BLADDER

- DAY-TIME
- Is the storage of urine
- NIGHT-TIME

Bladder is the organ similar to the "Official in Charge of Reservoir" and is responsible for accumulation and discharge of liquids through Qi transformation

More storing and less discharging, depending kidney Qi's nourishing

SAN JIAO

- DAY-TIME
- Is the pathway of the body fluid
- NIGHT-TIME

San Jiao is the organ similar to the "Official in Charge of Dredging" and is responsible for regulating water passage. San Jiao dominates Qi and transportation of body fluid bases on transformation of San Jiao's Qi

Being nourished by Body Fluid and Blood along with storing Qi in Body Fluid and Blood for daytime use

51

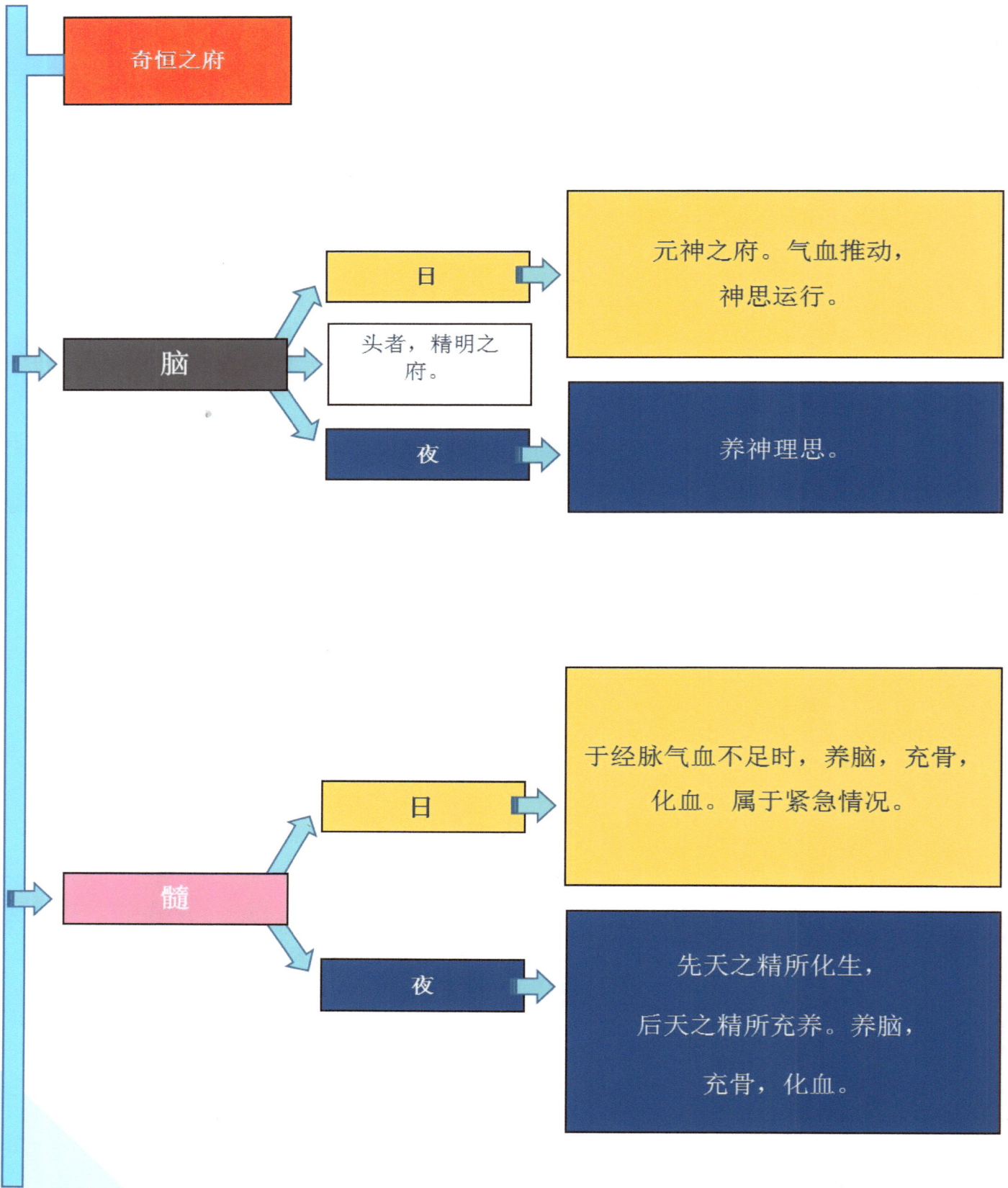

奇恒之府

脑

日 → 元神之府。气血推动，神思运行。

头者，精明之府。

夜 → 养神理思。

髓

日 → 于经脉气血不足时，养脑，充骨，化血。属于紧急情况。

夜 → 先天之精所化生，后天之精所充养。养脑，充骨，化血。

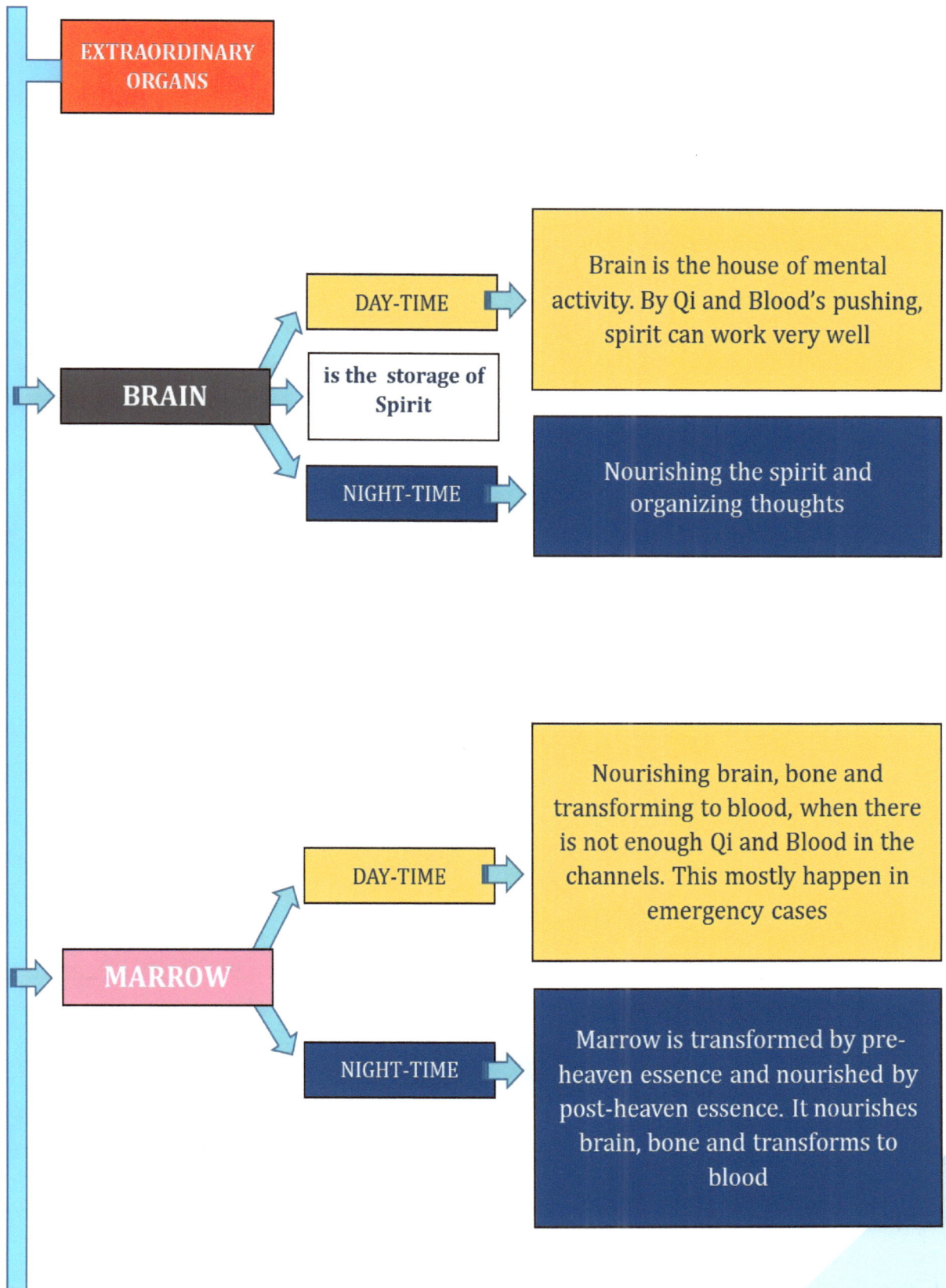

EXTRAORDINARY ORGANS

BRAIN

is the storage of Spirit

DAY-TIME → Brain is the house of mental activity. By Qi and Blood's pushing, spirit can work very well

NIGHT-TIME → Nourishing the spirit and organizing thoughts

MARROW

DAY-TIME → Nourishing brain, bone and transforming to blood, when there is not enough Qi and Blood in the channels. This mostly happen in emergency cases

NIGHT-TIME → Marrow is transformed by pre-heaven essence and nourished by post-heaven essence. It nourishes brain, bone and transforms to blood

53

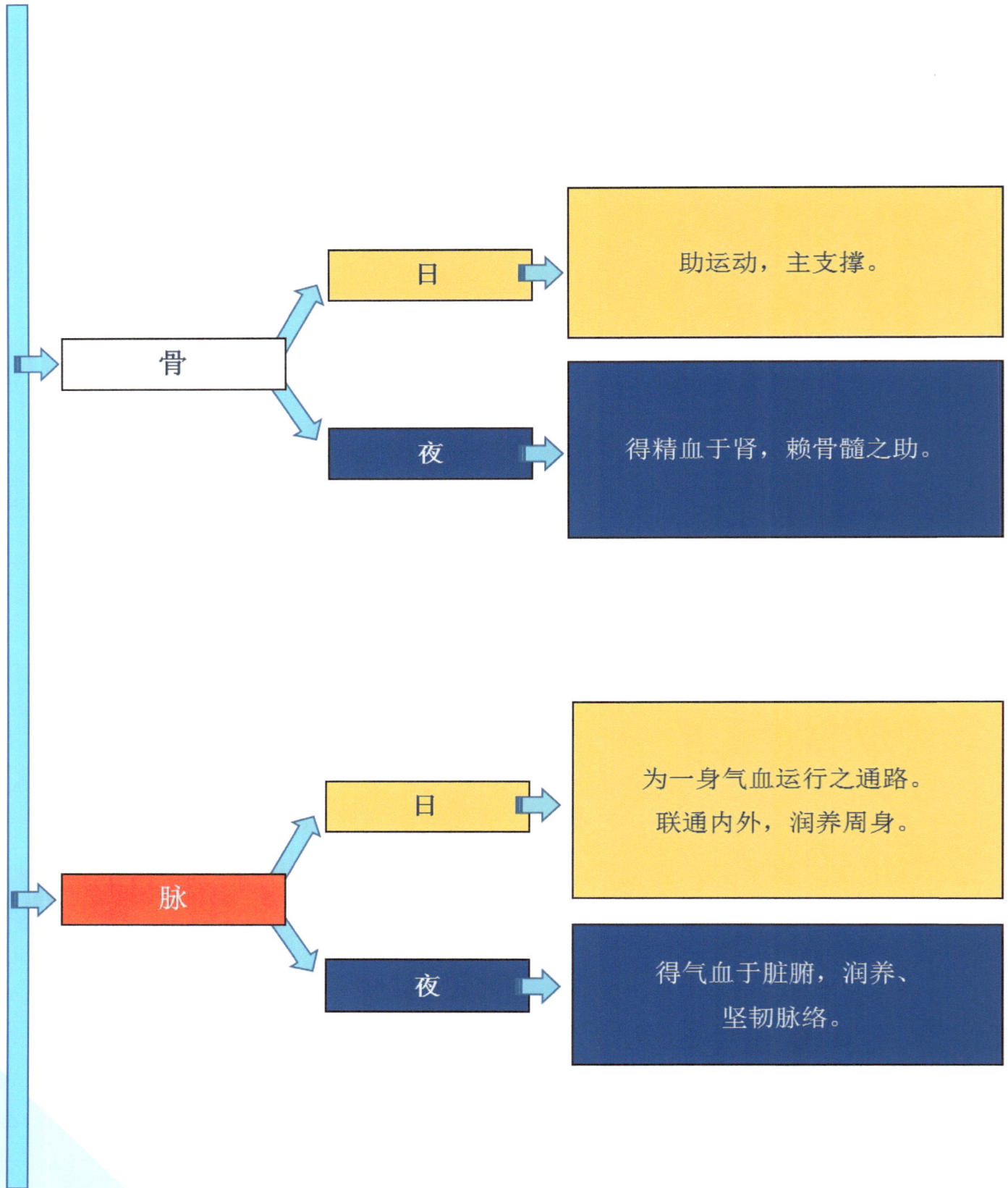

骨

日 → 助运动，主支撑。

夜 → 得精血于肾，赖骨髓之助。

脉

日 → 为一身气血运行之通路。
联通内外，润养周身。

夜 → 得气血于脏腑，润养、
坚韧脉络。

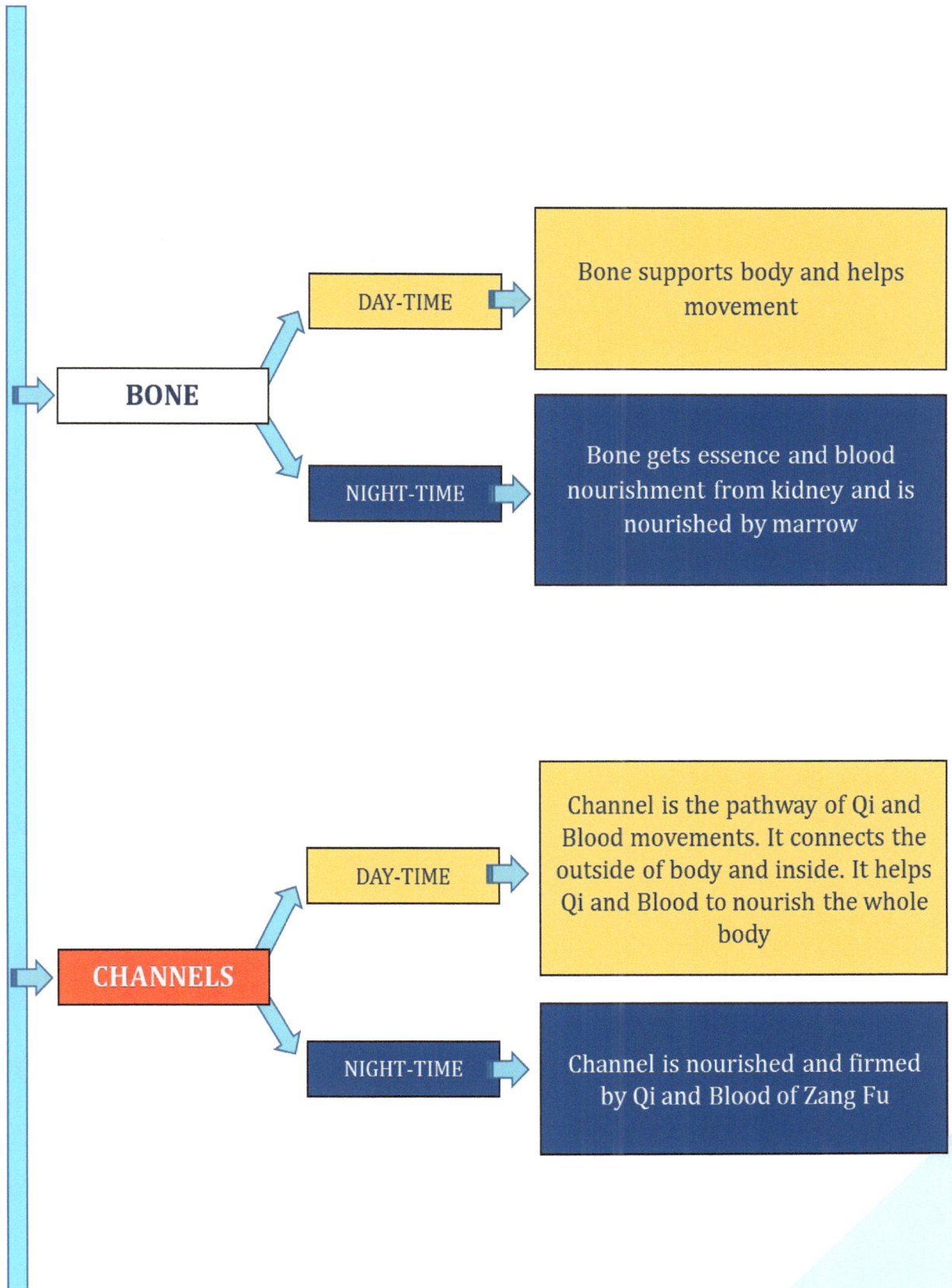

BONE

DAY-TIME → Bone supports body and helps movement

NIGHT-TIME → Bone gets essence and blood nourishment from kidney and is nourished by marrow

CHANNELS

DAY-TIME → Channel is the pathway of Qi and Blood movements. It connects the outside of body and inside. It helps Qi and Blood to nourish the whole body

NIGHT-TIME → Channel is nourished and firmed by Qi and Blood of Zang Fu

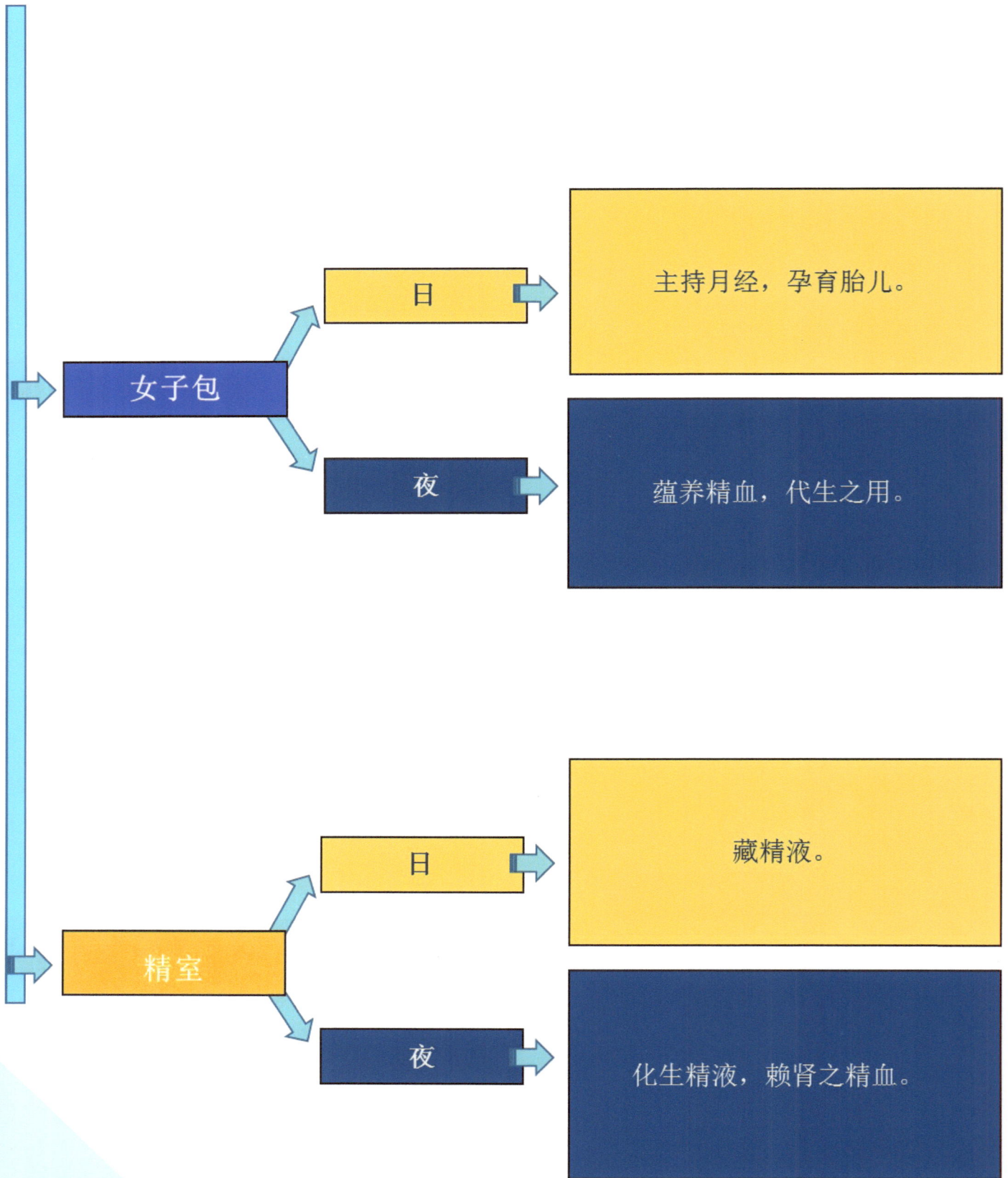

女子包

日 → 主持月经，孕育胎儿。

夜 → 蕴养精血，代生之用。

精室

日 → 藏精液。

夜 → 化生精液，赖肾之精血。

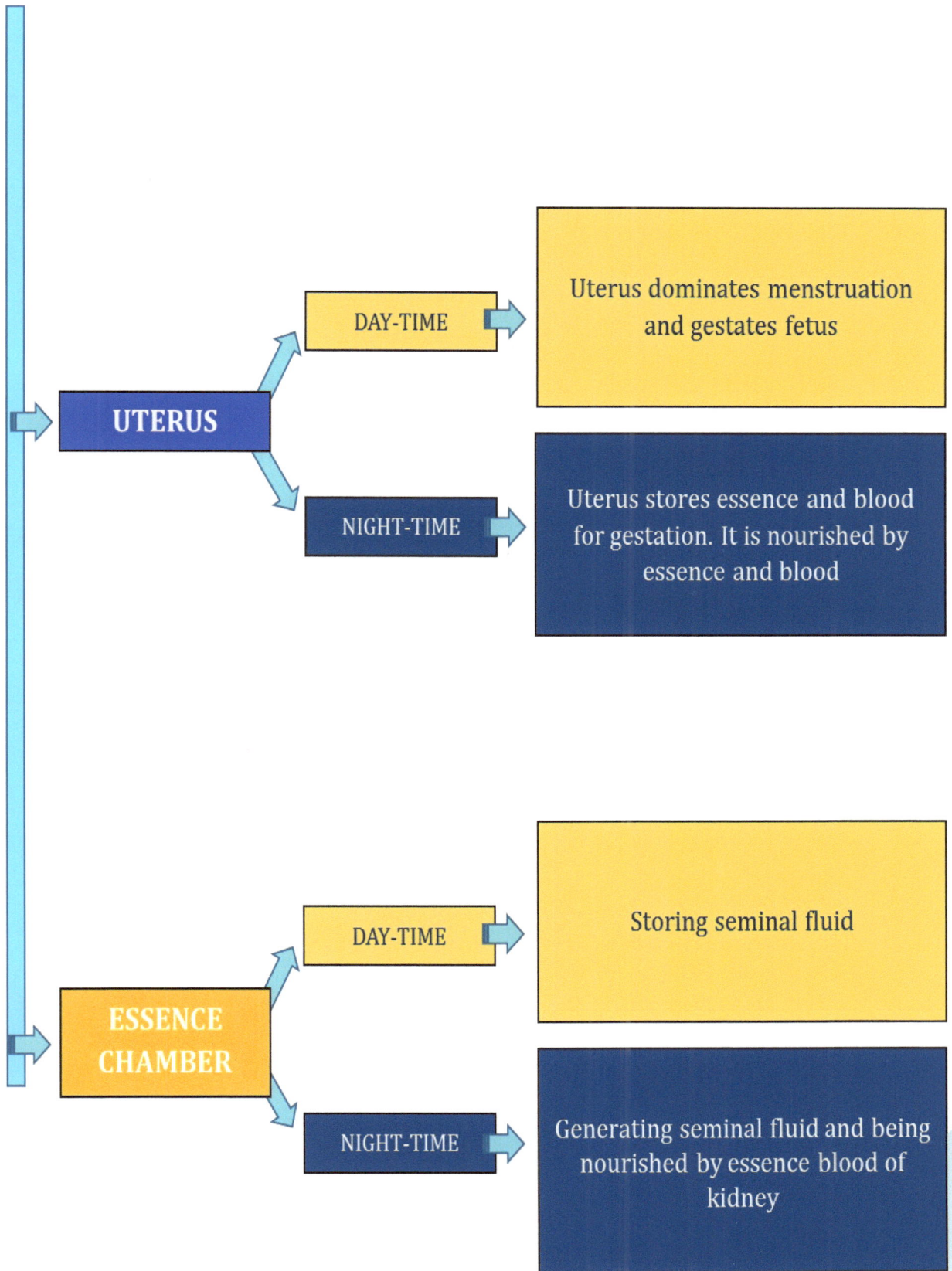

UTERUS

- DAY-TIME → Uterus dominates menstruation and gestates fetus
- NIGHT-TIME → Uterus stores essence and blood for gestation. It is nourished by essence and blood

ESSENCE CHAMBER

- DAY-TIME → Storing seminal fluid
- NIGHT-TIME → Generating seminal fluid and being nourished by essence blood of kidney

57

3.4气血津液理论的双极表现

气属阳，血和津液属阴。所以受到阴阳夜伏昼出规律的影响，气血津液也遵循这一规律。但是气血津液在夜间并非完全意义的潜伏不动，而是运行相对于日间来说变得十分缓慢。同时由于气血津液自身的特殊性质，其日夜的双极表现又有它们自身的特点。

日间，气温煦和推动血液和津液运行，并且统摄血液、津液在其各自的通道中流行。同时，日间我们所食入的各种食物经由脾胃的运化转变为谷气。再部分转化为血液和津液以补充它们的不足。

3.4. The Manifestation of the Two Opposite Theory of Qi, Blood and Body Fluid

Qi belongs to Yang. Blood and body fluid belong to Yin. Influenced by the rule of Yin and Yang, daytime being very active and the night being hidden, qi, blood and body fluid also follow this rule. However, qi, blood and body fluid are not completely hiding motionless in the nighttime. They just run relatively slow compared to the day. Qi, blood and body fluid has its own characteristics and manifestation within the Two Opposite Theory.

In the daytime Qi warms and pushes blood and body fluid circulation. It governs blood and body fluid circulating in their pathways. At the same time, all the foods what we eat are transformed into Grain Qi by spleen and stomach. Grain Qi changes to blood and body fluid. This process can provide the supply of blood and body fluid for consumption.

夜间，气的流动变得缓慢，血液和津液流动也随之变得缓慢。同时，血液和津液开始反过来补养气在日间的消耗。使其有足够的能量在次日继续工作。

气血津液的这种日夜转化规律，我称之为气血津液理论的双极表现。

In the nighttime, qi moves slowly causing the movement of blood and body fluid to slow down. During this time, blood and body fluid start to nourish Qi for next day's work.

The day and night transformation rule of Qi, Blood and Body Fluid is named the Manifestation of the Two Opposite Theory of Qi, Blood and Body Fluid.

3.5 经络理论的双极表现

十二经络和奇经八脉为人体经络系统的主干。而其他诸如络脉、孙络、浮络、经筋和皮部等等则为经脉不同级别的分支。但是不管是主干还是分支，它们赖以工作的基础是其内部流行的气血。所以，经络内气血的不同状态决定了经络在工作中的不同表现。而气血的运行大体以阴阳的夜伏昼出规律为基础。所以，经络运行的规律同样在大体上遵循夜伏昼出的规律。只在个别经脉上有所不同，如下：

3.5. The Manifestation of the Two Opposite Theory of Jing Luo

Twelve meridians and eight extra meridians are trunks of the meridian system. The other channels such as; Luo Connecting channels, Superficial collaterals, Minute collaterals, Muscle meridians, Cutaneous regions and so on are different level branches of the main meridians. Both the trunks and branches of the meridians depend upon Qi and Blood passing through the meridians for their basic functions. Therefore, differential status of Qi and Blood in meridians will decide the working manifestations of meridians. The operation of Qi and Blood are generally based on the rule of Yin and Yang with the daytime being very active and the night being hidden. Therefore, the functionality and operation of meridians are generally based on the same rule. There are some differences and exceptions on several meridians.

肾经、冲脉和任督二脉由于协助肾脏平衡人体的阴阳，促进阴阳的转化。所以它们在功能上的特点与肾脏的双极表现一致。

The characteristics and function of Kidney meridian, Penetrating vessel, Conception vessel and Governing vessel are the same as the manifestation of the Two Opposite Theory of kidney. These meridians support kidney to balance Yin and Yang of human body and improve the inter-transformation between Yin and Yang.

3.6疾病的双极表现

　　疾病同于天地万物。所以它们同样遵守世间阴阳转化的基本规律，即夜伏昼出。但是，凡事皆有特例。就好像，社会中并非所有人都是日出而作，日落而息一样。疾病中也有许多是反其道而行之的。但是不管正反，它们始终会呈现阴和阳，日和夜的双极表现。既然有迹可循，自然有法可依，必然有计可施。所以古人经常说的"师法自然"其实是放至五湖四海皆准的至理。

3.6. The Manifestation of the Two Opposite Theory of Diseases

Diseases are the same as everything else in the world. They follow the same rule of Yin and Yang with the daytime being very active and the night being hidden. With that being said there are exceptions, some of diseases act in a diametrically opposed manner. Regardless of positive or negative, they still appear with the manifestation of Two Opposite Theory of Yin and Yang and daytime-nighttime. There are some indications which can be tracked. There must be laws for people to follow, and ways for people to use those laws. That is why the ancients always said it is best to learn from nature, because it is the reflection of the whole world.

综上所述，我们可以发现，双极表现虽然大体表现为夜伏昼出。但并非单纯的教条的夜伏昼出那么简单。它更深层的含义是对人体和疾病在昼夜这两个极端的时间段中所表现出的性质完全不同的，甚至相反的功能和现象的总结。

From the above, we could find that the manifestation of Two Opposite appears generally as nighttime hidden and daytime active. But it is not quite that simple of a doctrine. It has a deeper meaning. It is the summary of the features and phenomenon which come from the total different or opposite manifestation of human body and diseases while shown in these two extreme periods of day and night.

4. 双极治则

以日夜分治为主要特点，包括基本治则和联合治则两部分。

4.1基本治则

包括理、化、养三种基本治则。

4.1.1 理法

理，为梳理，调和的意思。此种治则重在疏导、整理、调和人体各部及各部之间的关系，治法平和。

4. The Therapeutic Principles of the Two Opposites

Treatment is separated by characteristics of daytime and nighttime. It includes the basic therapeutic principles and the united therapeutic principles two parts.

4.1. The Basic Therapeutic Principles

Regulation, resolving and improvement are the three basic therapeutic principles.

4.1.1. Regulation

Regulation means an orderly flow and reconciliation. This therapeutic principle focuses on dislodging, systemizing and reconciliation the relationship of different parts of human body. It is mild and gentle.

4.1.2 化法

化，为化解的意思。此种方法源于理法，但是更加积极。此种治则重在使用强力手段破解、驱散和消除致病因素，治法猛烈。

4.1.3 养法

等同于传统意义的补法。此种治则重在补充人体各部及各部之间的不足。

72

4.1.2. Resolving

Resolving means transforming and disintegrating. It comes from Regulation, but more active. Resolving focuses on using strong treatment to break, dispel and eliminate pathogenic factors. Therefore, it can be violent.

4.1.3. Improvement

Improvement is the same as tonification or nourishing in traditional method. It is focuses on tonifying and nourishing different parts of human body along with the tissues between these parts.

4.2联合治则

包括日间治则和夜间治则。

4.2.1 日间治则

当疾病的发展规律和患者的生活规律均遵循阴阳昼夜变化规律的时候，日间治则以理法、化法为主，养法为辅。当疾病的发展规律和患者的生活规律与阴阳昼夜变化规律相反的时候，日间治则采用理法、化法和养法份量相等的配比规律。

4.2. The Associated Therapeutic Principles

The Associated Therapeutic Principles includes Daytime Therapeutic Principles and Nighttime Therapeutic Principles.

4.2.1. Daytime Therapeutic Principles

When the development rules of diseases and the daily life of patients follows the day and night transformation rules of Yin and Yang, the Daytime Therapeutic Principles focus on Regulation and Resolving supported by Improvement. However, when development rules of diseases and daily life of the patient are contrary to the day and night transformation, Daytime Therapeutic Principles adopt the matching rule of equal proportion between Regulation or Resolving and Improvement.

4.2.2 夜间治则

当疾病的发展规律和患者的生活规律均遵循阴阳昼夜变化规律的时候，夜间治则以养法为主，理法、化法为辅。当疾病的发展规律和患者的生活规律与阴阳昼夜变化规律相反的时候，夜间治则分为缓急两方面。如果病情紧急，症状严重。夜间治则以理法、化法为主，养法为辅；如果病情缓和，症状缠绵。夜间治则采用理法、化法和养法份量相当或理法、化法略重于养法的配比规律。

4.2.2. Nighttime Therapeutic Principles

When development rules of diseases and daily life of the patient follow the day and night transformation rules of Yin and Yang, Nighttime Therapeutic Principles focus on Improvement supported by Regulation and Resolving. However, when development rules of diseases and the daily life of the patient are contrary to day and night transformation rule, Nighttime Therapeutic Principles are separated into easy and urgent aspects. If the disease is an emergency and with severe symptoms the Nighttime Therapeutic Principles focuses on Regulation and Resolving supported by Improvement. Whereas, if the disease is moderate with lingering symptoms the Nighttime Therapeutic Principles adopt the matching rule of equal proportion between Regulation or Resolving and Improvement. Sometimes the matching rule of proportion results with Regulation or Resolving being stronger or more evident than Improvement.

下面我将双极治则分阴阳、脏腑、气血津液三部分简述，希望给初学者一些指导和建议。但是需要注意的是，以下所有简述双极治则，只作为临床治疗时的一种辅助参考手段。它们不能被原封不动地照搬，而是应该在辨证论治的基础上，参考变化，这才是它存在的意义。

In the following discussions, I will separate the Therapeutic Principles of the Two Opposites Theory of Yin and Yang, Zang Fu and Qi, Blood and Body Fluid into three parts discussing them in a simple manner. I hope to give beginners some guidance and advice. It is important to note that all of the following brief descriptions of the Therapeutic Principles of the Two Opposite Theory is only to be utilized as an auxiliary reference means of clinical treatment. They cannot be copied exactly, but should change based on the syndrome differentiation. This is a significant element of the theory.

4.2.3 阴阳双极治则简述

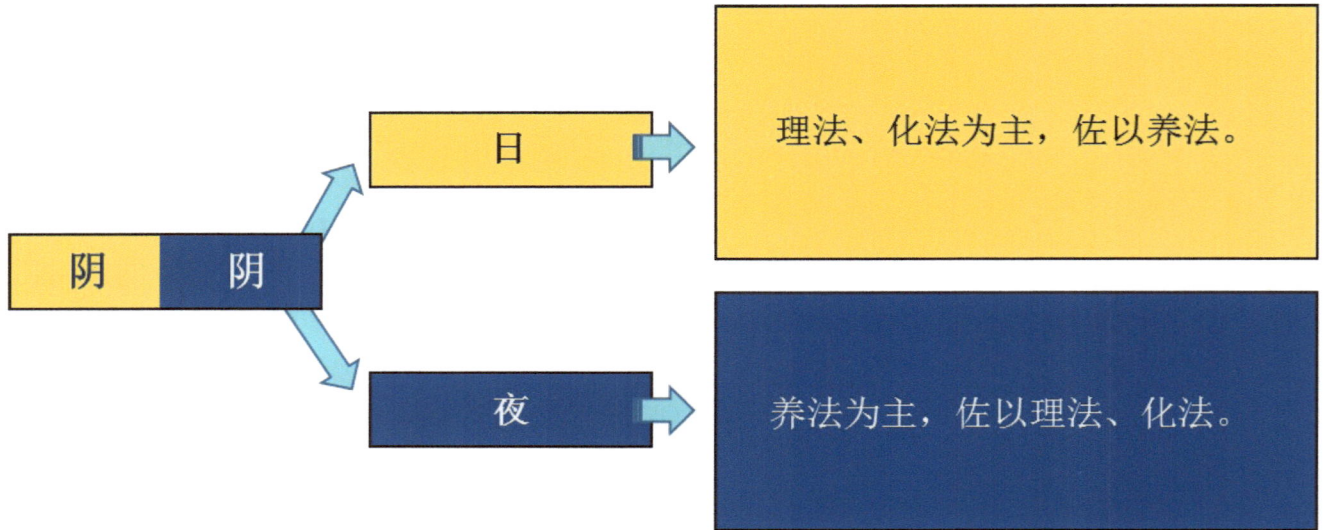

日	理法、化法为主，佐以养法。
夜	养法为主，佐以理法、化法。

阴 阴

4.2.3. Brief Description of the Yin Yang Therapeutic Principles of the Two Opposites

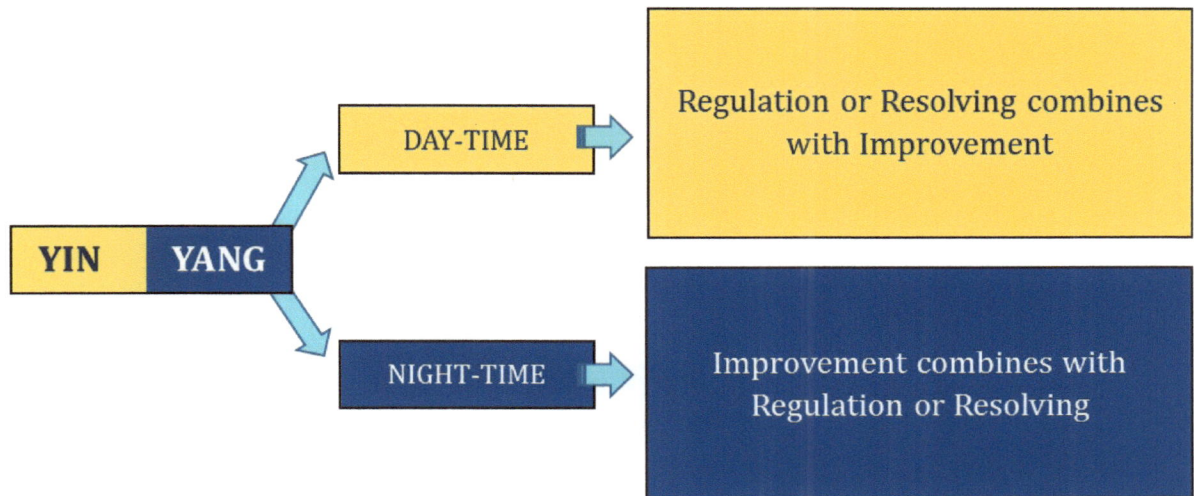

4.2.4 脏腑双极治则简述

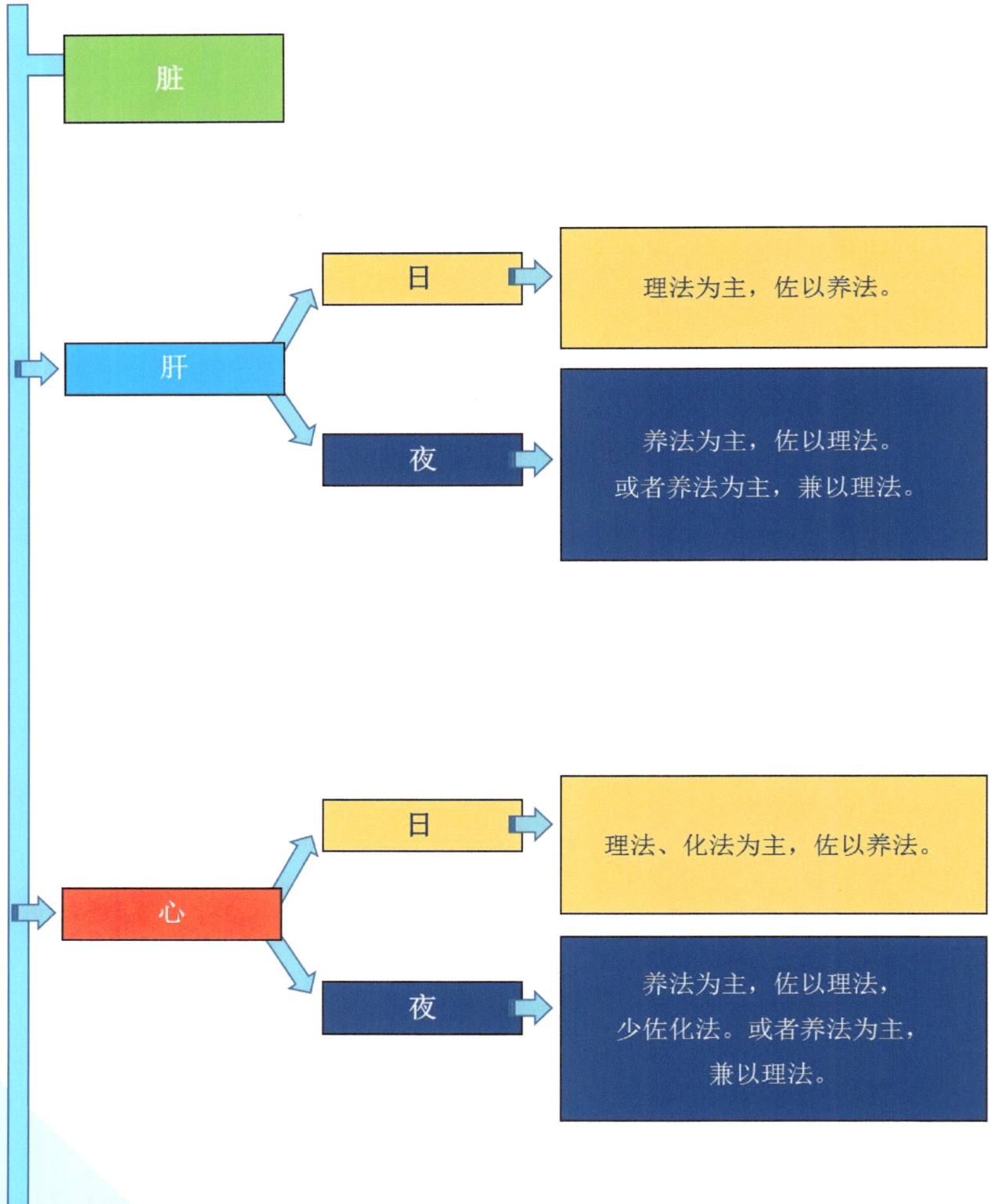

脏

肝

日 → 理法为主，佐以养法。

夜 → 养法为主，佐以理法。
或者养法为主，兼以理法。

心

日 → 理法、化法为主，佐以养法。

夜 → 养法为主，佐以理法，
少佐化法。或者养法为主，
兼以理法。

4.2.4. Brief Description of the Zang Fu Therapeutic Principles of the Two Opposites

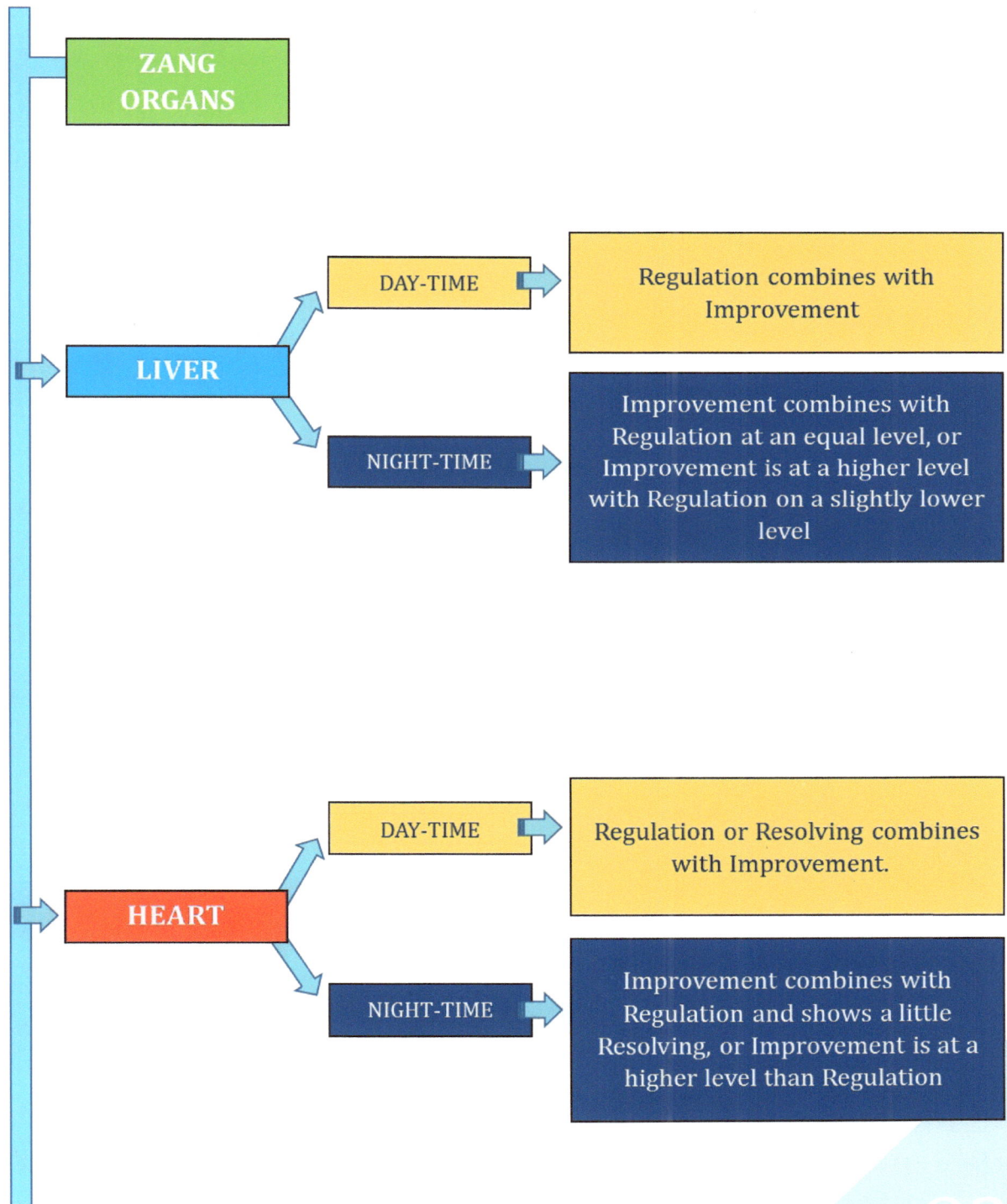

ZANG ORGANS

LIVER
- DAY-TIME → Regulation combines with Improvement
- NIGHT-TIME → Improvement combines with Regulation at an equal level, or Improvement is at a higher level with Regulation on a slightly lower level

HEART
- DAY-TIME → Regulation or Resolving combines with Improvement.
- NIGHT-TIME → Improvement combines with Regulation and shows a little Resolving, or Improvement is at a higher level than Regulation

83

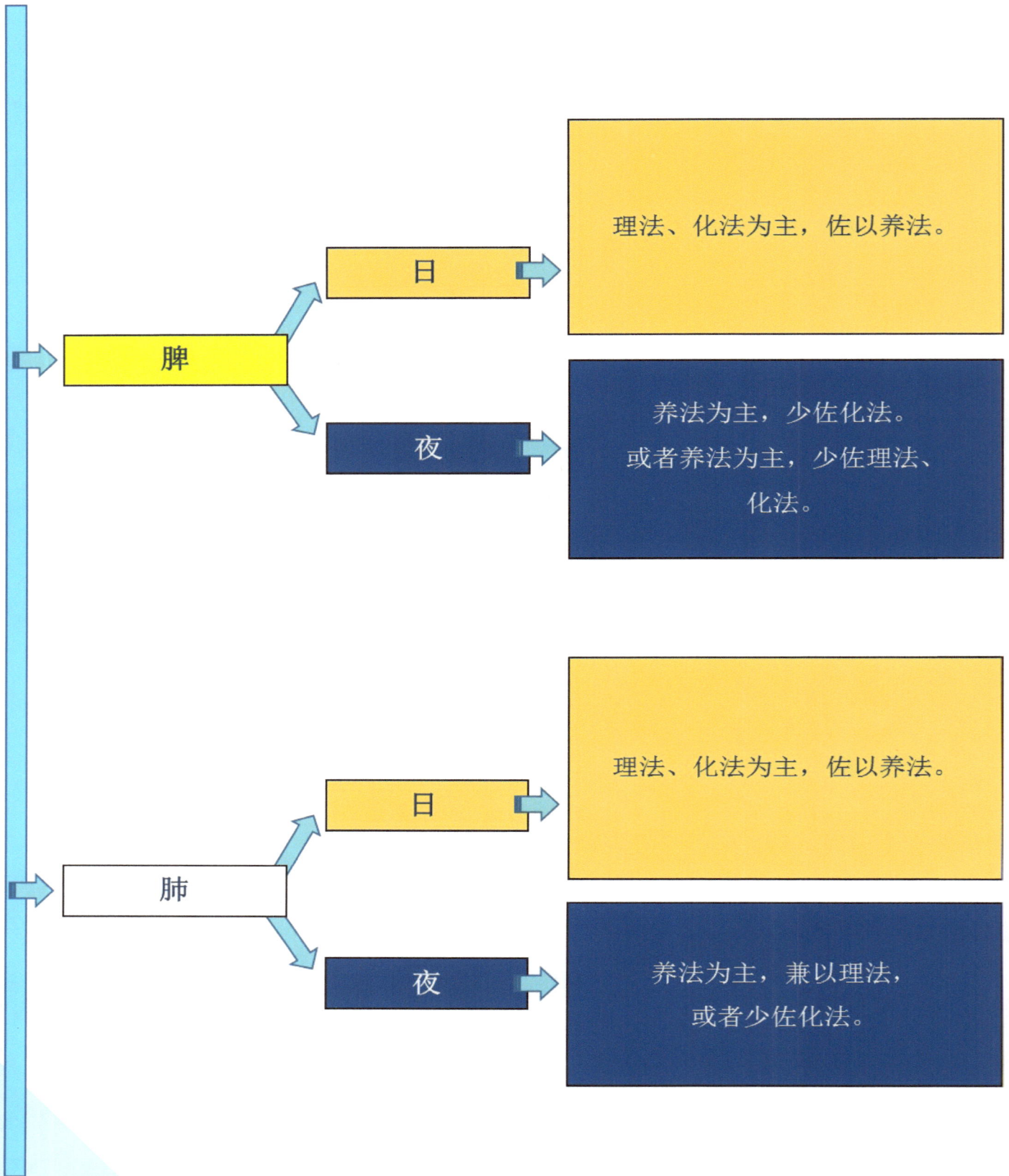

脾

日 → 理法、化法为主，佐以养法。

夜 → 养法为主，少佐化法。
或者养法为主，少佐理法、
化法。

肺

日 → 理法、化法为主，佐以养法。

夜 → 养法为主，兼以理法，
或者少佐化法。

84

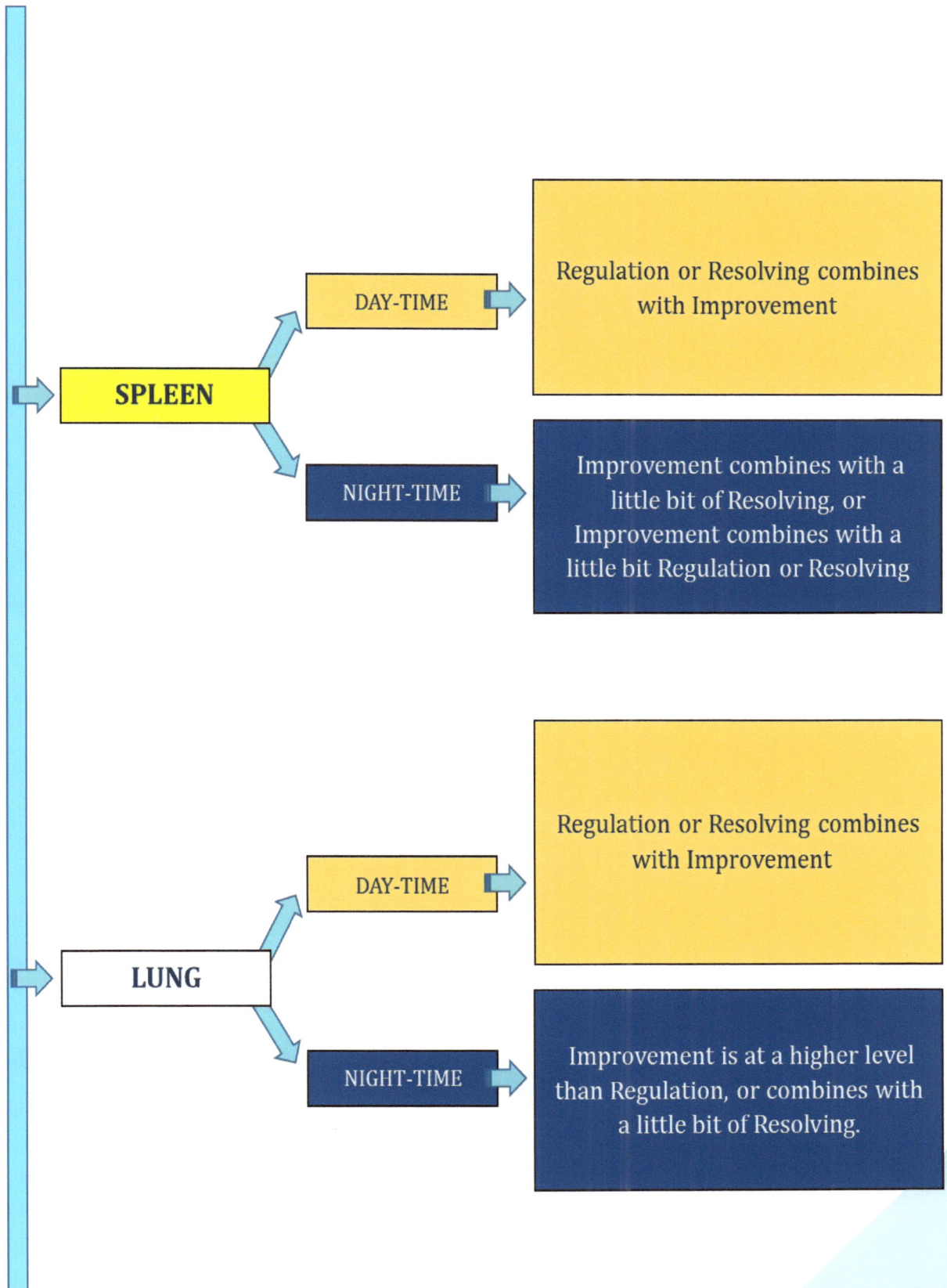

SPLEEN

DAY-TIME → Regulation or Resolving combines with Improvement

NIGHT-TIME → Improvement combines with a little bit of Resolving, or Improvement combines with a little bit Regulation or Resolving

LUNG

DAY-TIME → Regulation or Resolving combines with Improvement

NIGHT-TIME → Improvement is at a higher level than Regulation, or combines with a little bit of Resolving.

85

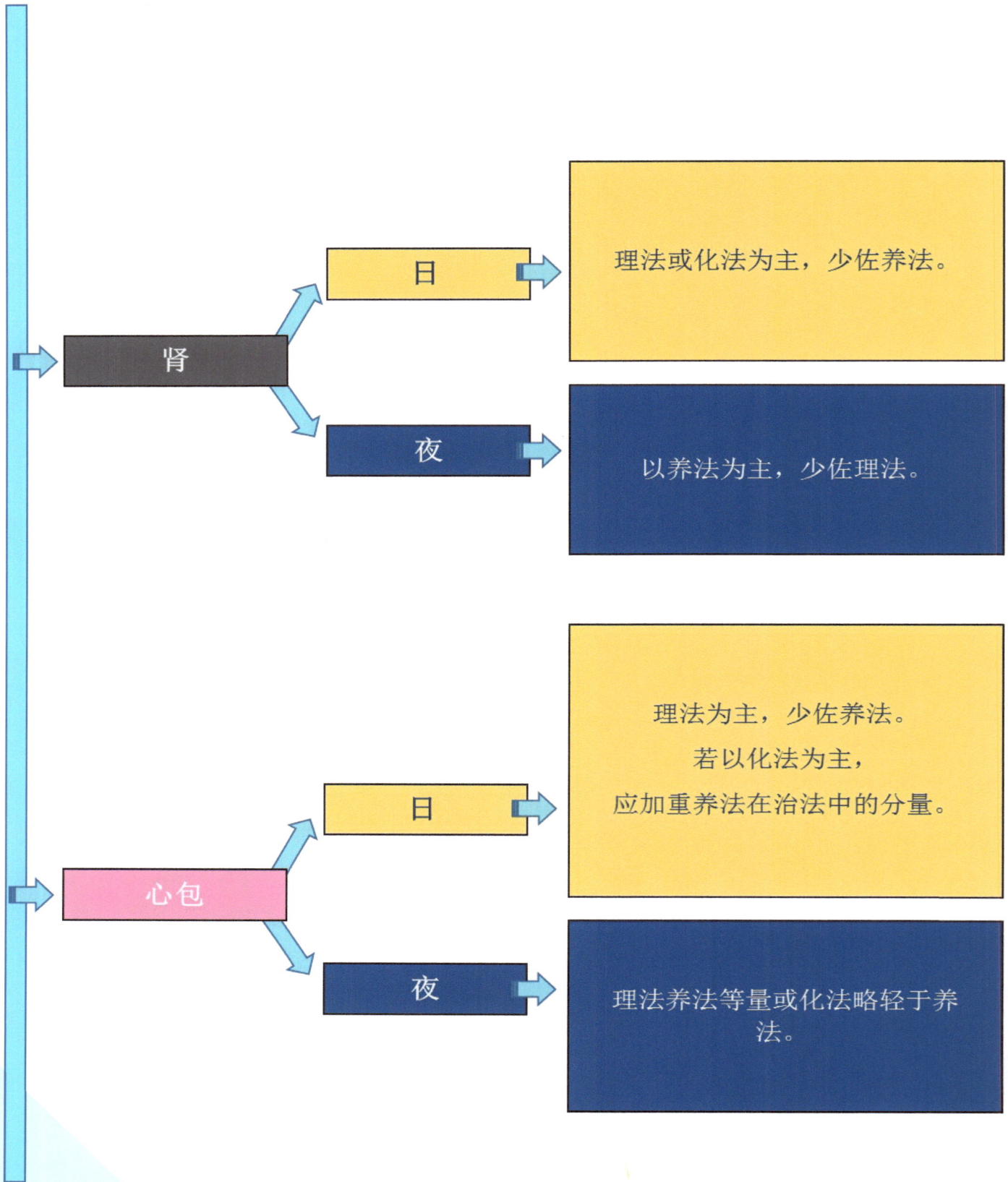

肾

日 → 理法或化法为主，少佐养法。

夜 → 以养法为主，少佐理法。

心包

日 → 理法为主，少佐养法。
若以化法为主，
应加重养法在治法中的分量。

夜 → 理法养法等量或化法略轻于养法。

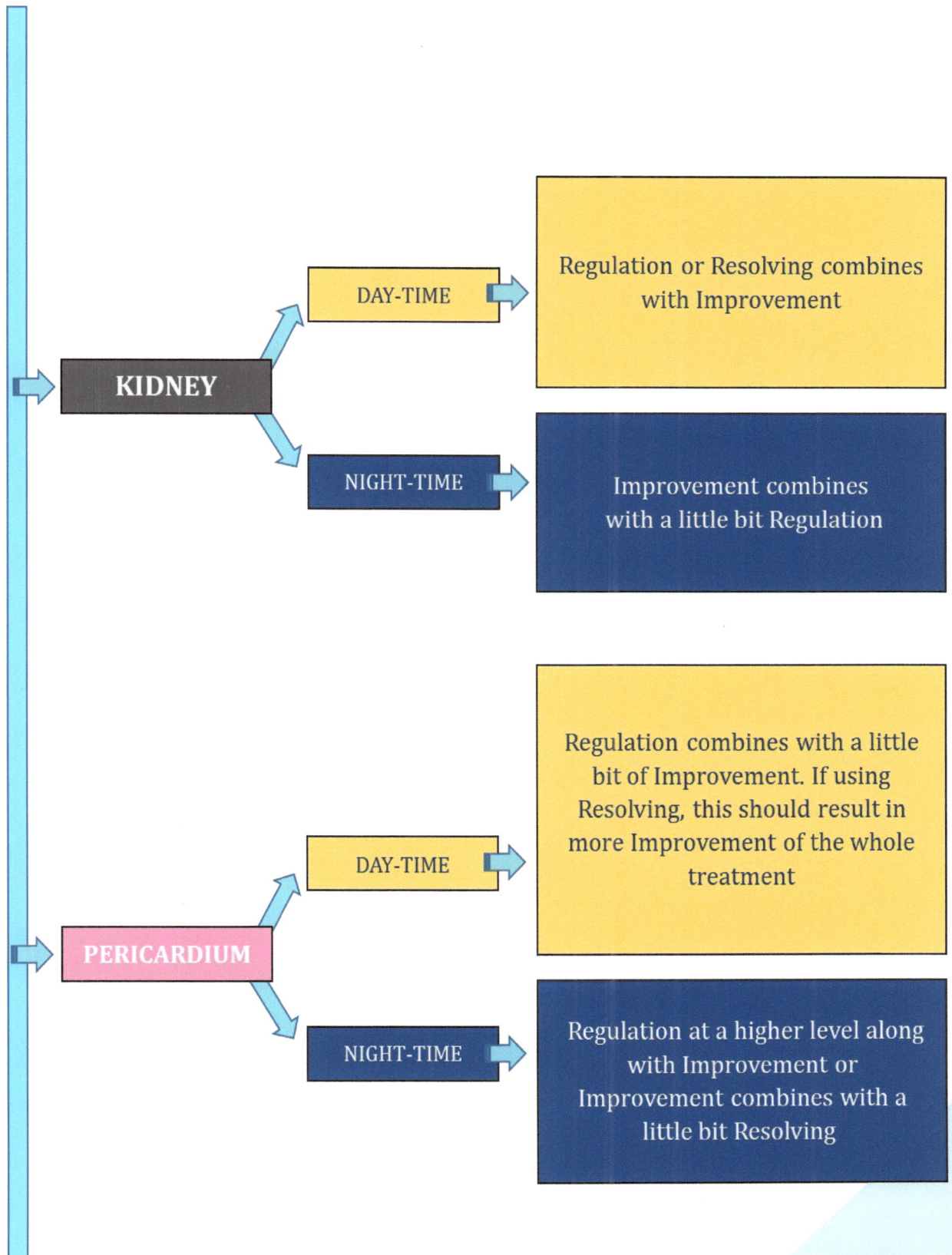

KIDNEY

DAY-TIME → Regulation or Resolving combines with Improvement

NIGHT-TIME → Improvement combines with a little bit Regulation

PERICARDIUM

DAY-TIME → Regulation combines with a little bit of Improvement. If using Resolving, this should result in more Improvement of the whole treatment

NIGHT-TIME → Regulation at a higher level along with Improvement or Improvement combines with a little bit Resolving

87

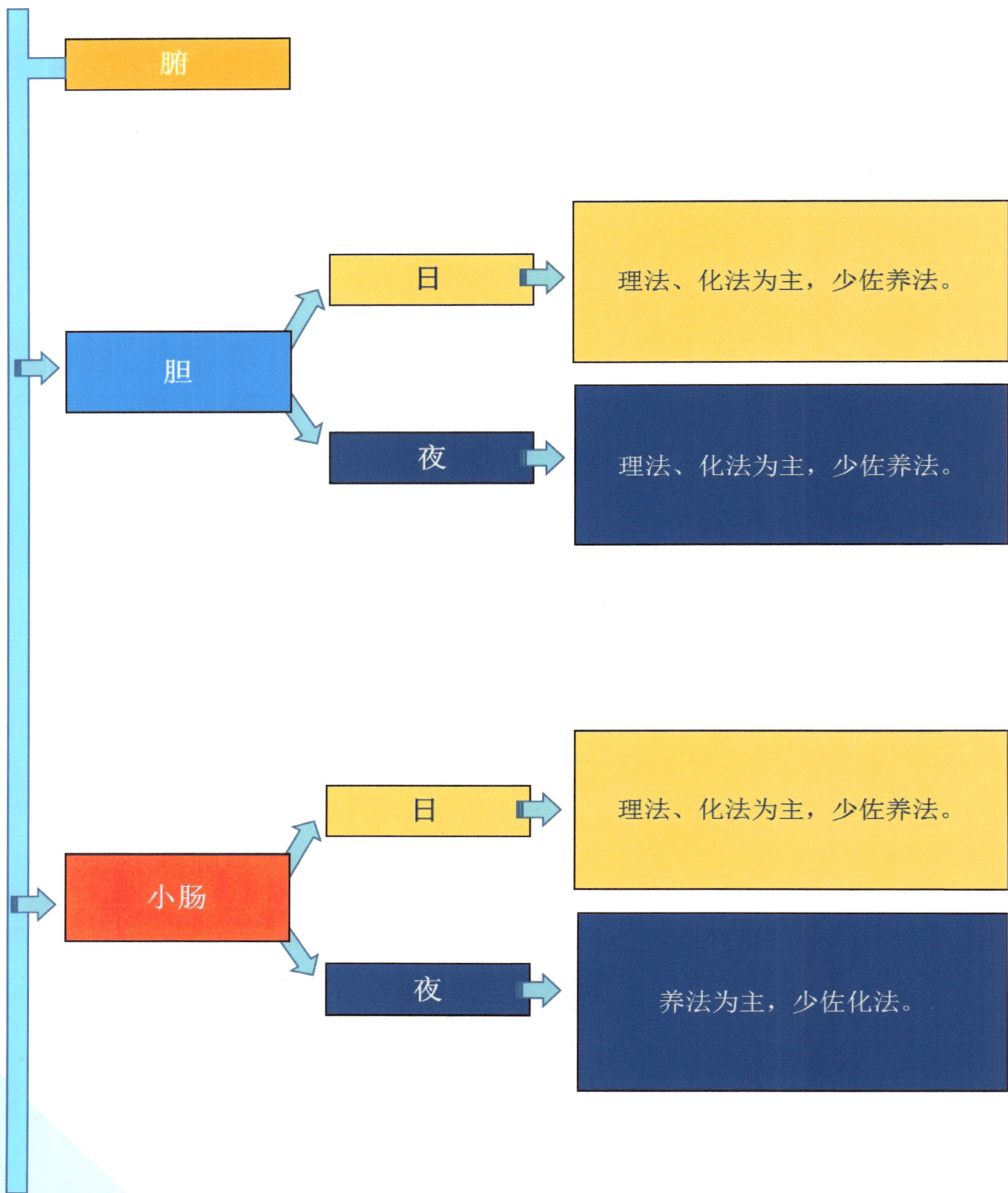

腑

胆

日 → 理法、化法为主，少佐养法。

夜 → 理法、化法为主，少佐养法。

小肠

日 → 理法、化法为主，少佐养法。

夜 → 养法为主，少佐化法。

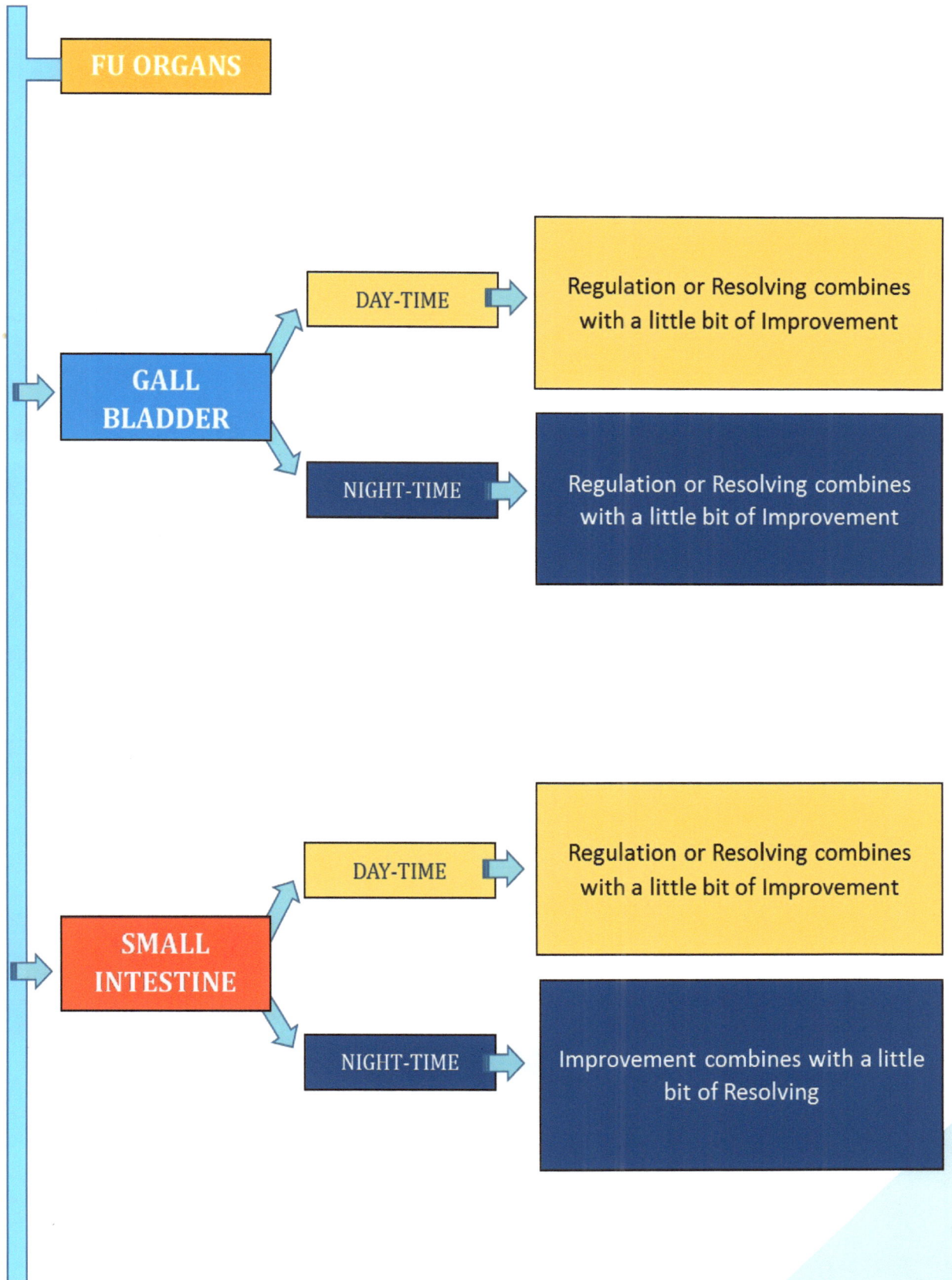

FU ORGANS

GALL BLADDER

DAY-TIME → Regulation or Resolving combines with a little bit of Improvement

NIGHT-TIME → Regulation or Resolving combines with a little bit of Improvement

SMALL INTESTINE

DAY-TIME → Regulation or Resolving combines with a little bit of Improvement

NIGHT-TIME → Improvement combines with a little bit of Resolving

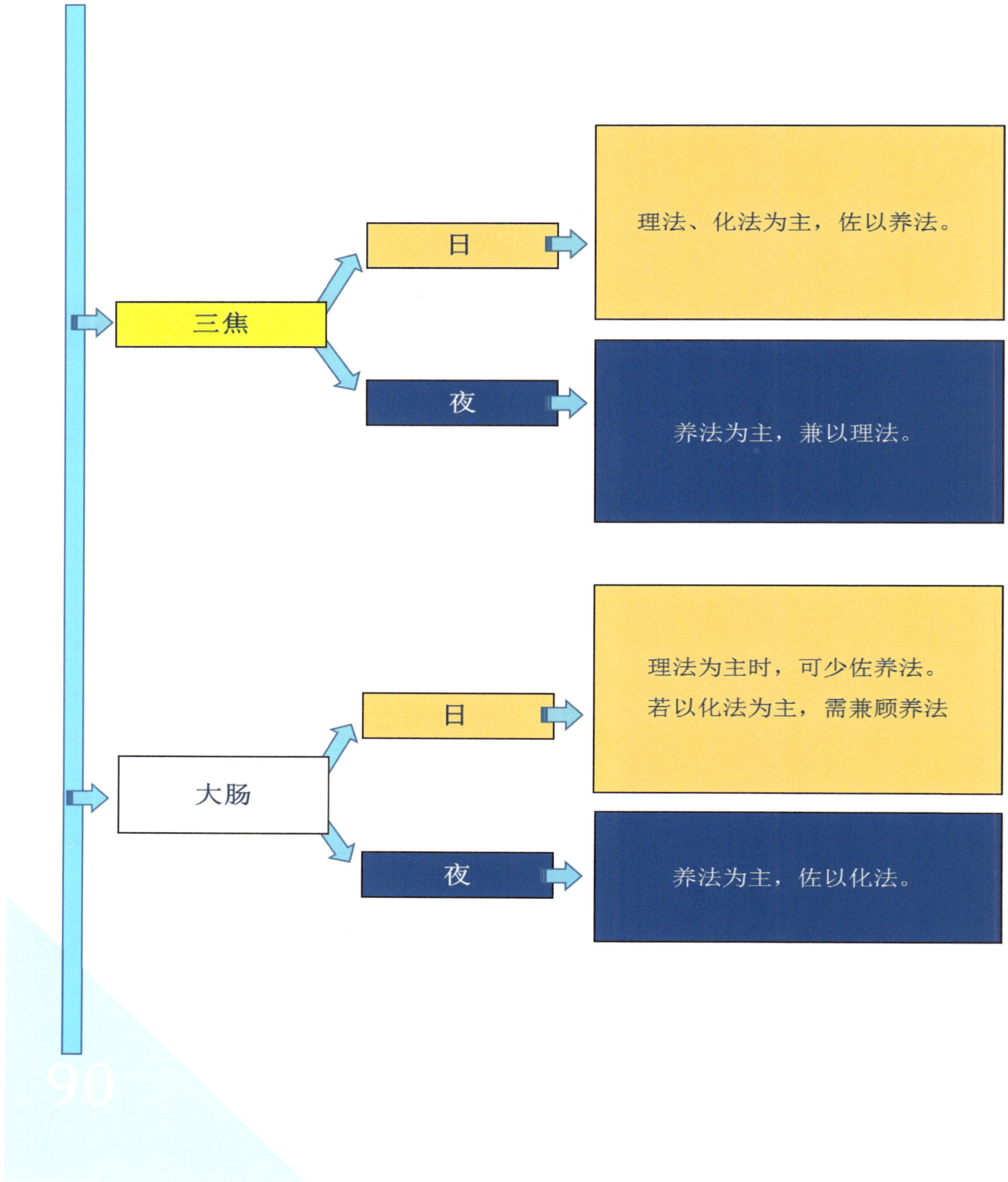

三焦

日 → 理法、化法为主，佐以养法。

夜 → 养法为主，兼以理法。

大肠

日 → 理法为主时，可少佐养法。
若以化法为主，需兼顾养法

夜 → 养法为主，佐以化法。

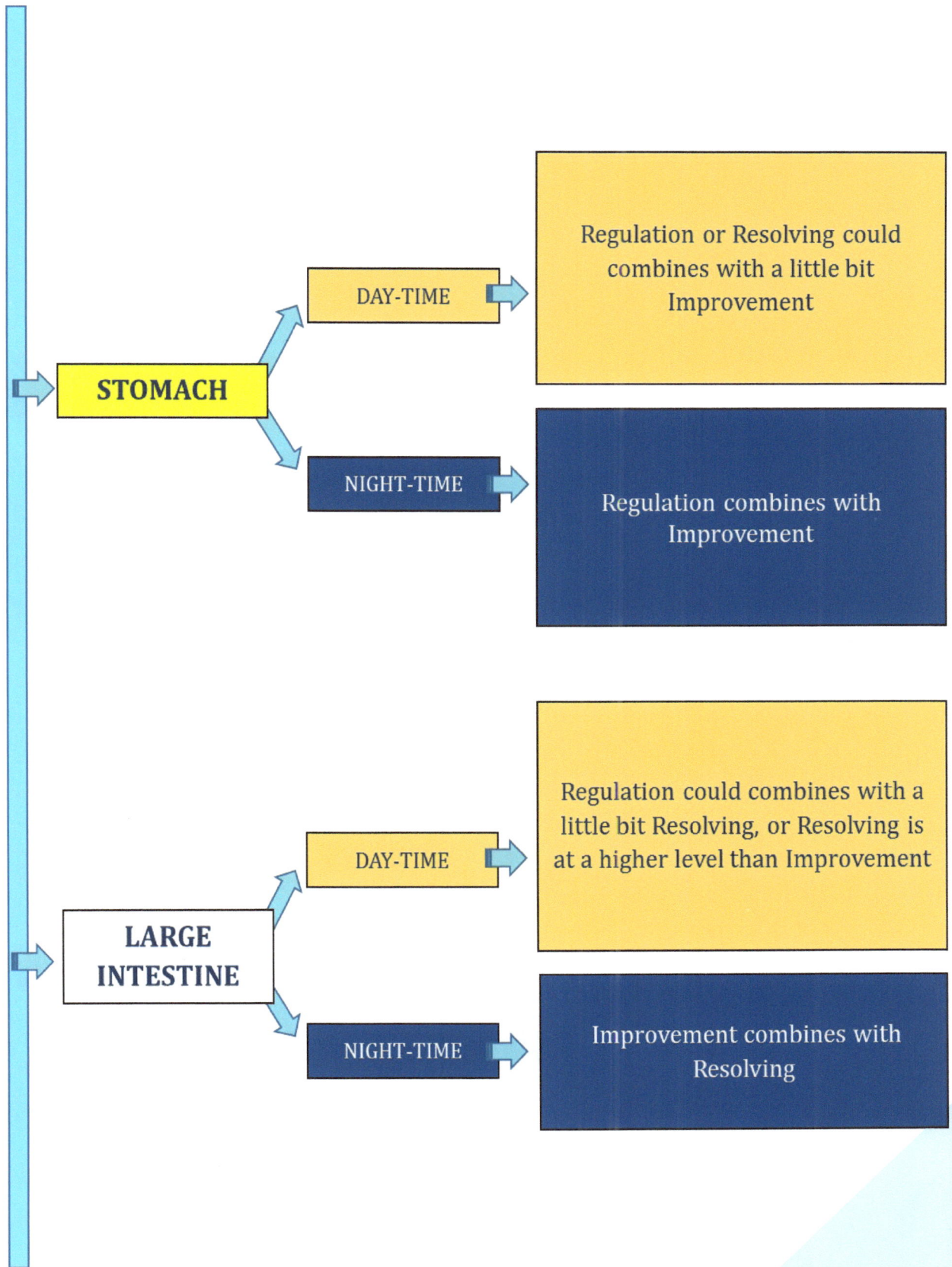

STOMACH

DAY-TIME → Regulation or Resolving could combines with a little bit Improvement

NIGHT-TIME → Regulation combines with Improvement

LARGE INTESTINE

DAY-TIME → Regulation could combines with a little bit Resolving, or Resolving is at a higher level than Improvement

NIGHT-TIME → Improvement combines with Resolving

91

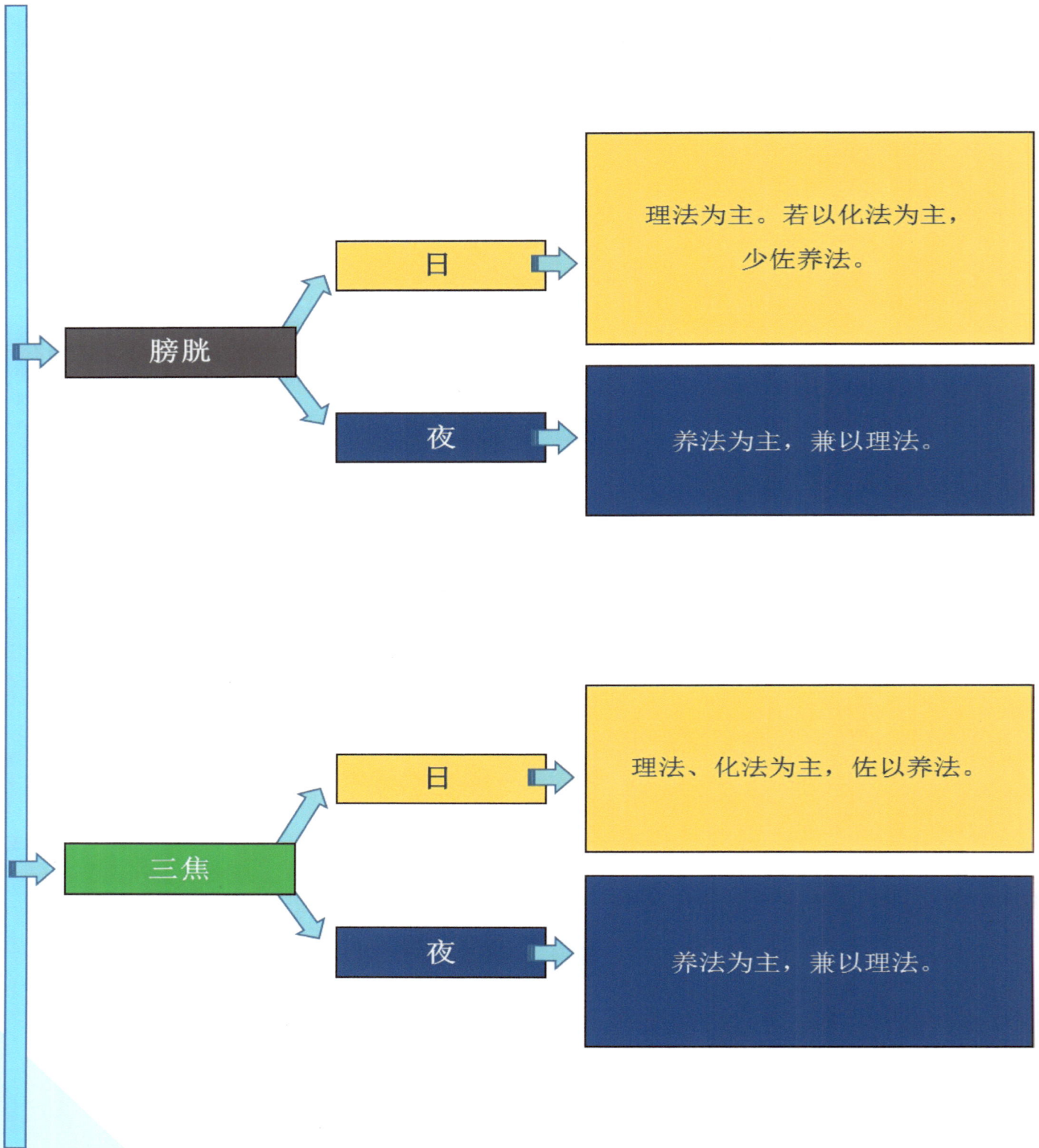

膀胱

日 → 理法为主。若以化法为主，少佐养法。

夜 → 养法为主，兼以理法。

三焦

日 → 理法、化法为主，佐以养法。

夜 → 养法为主，兼以理法。

92

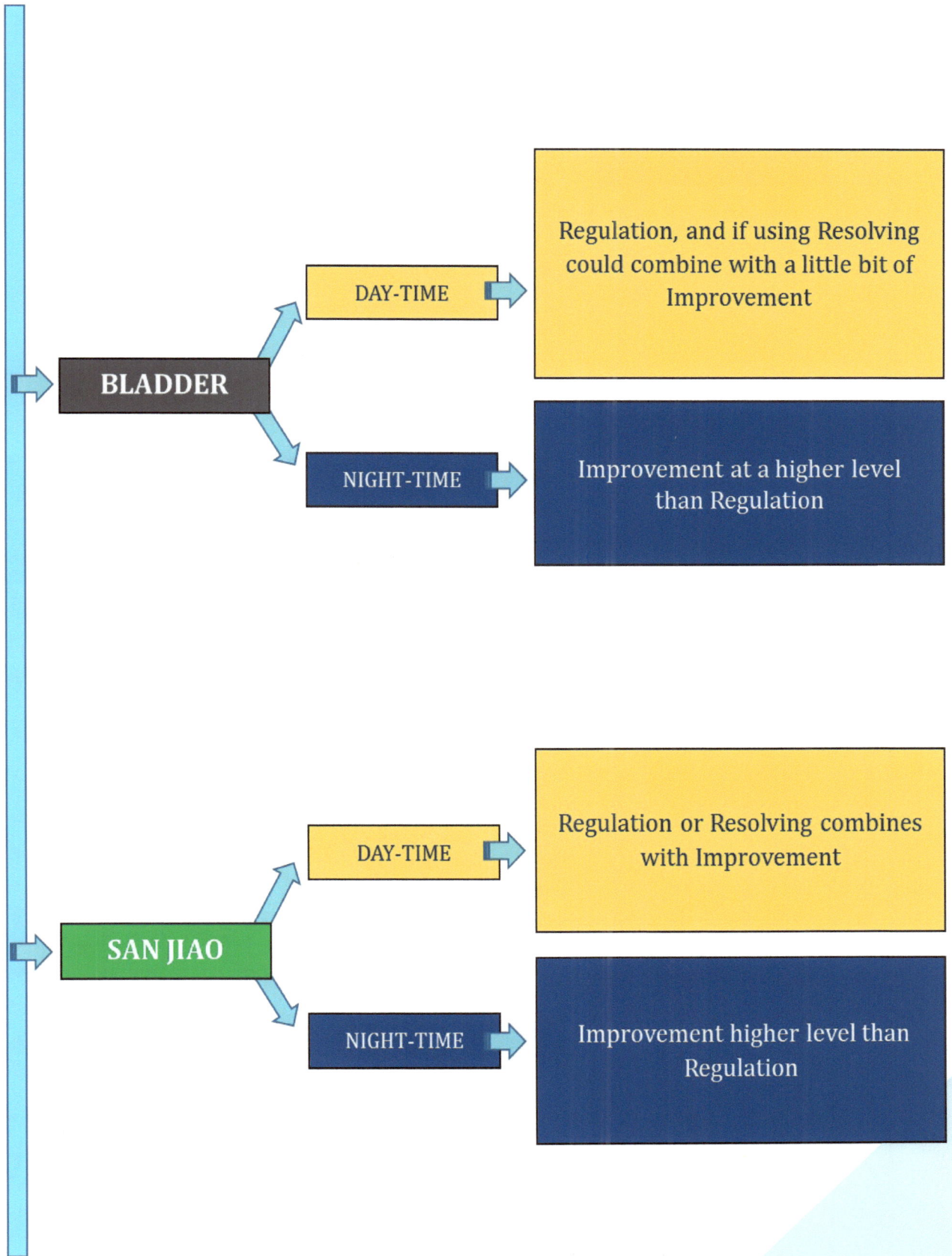

BLADDER

DAY-TIME → Regulation, and if using Resolving could combine with a little bit of Improvement

NIGHT-TIME → Improvement at a higher level than Regulation

SAN JIAO

DAY-TIME → Regulation or Resolving combines with Improvement

NIGHT-TIME → Improvement higher level than Regulation

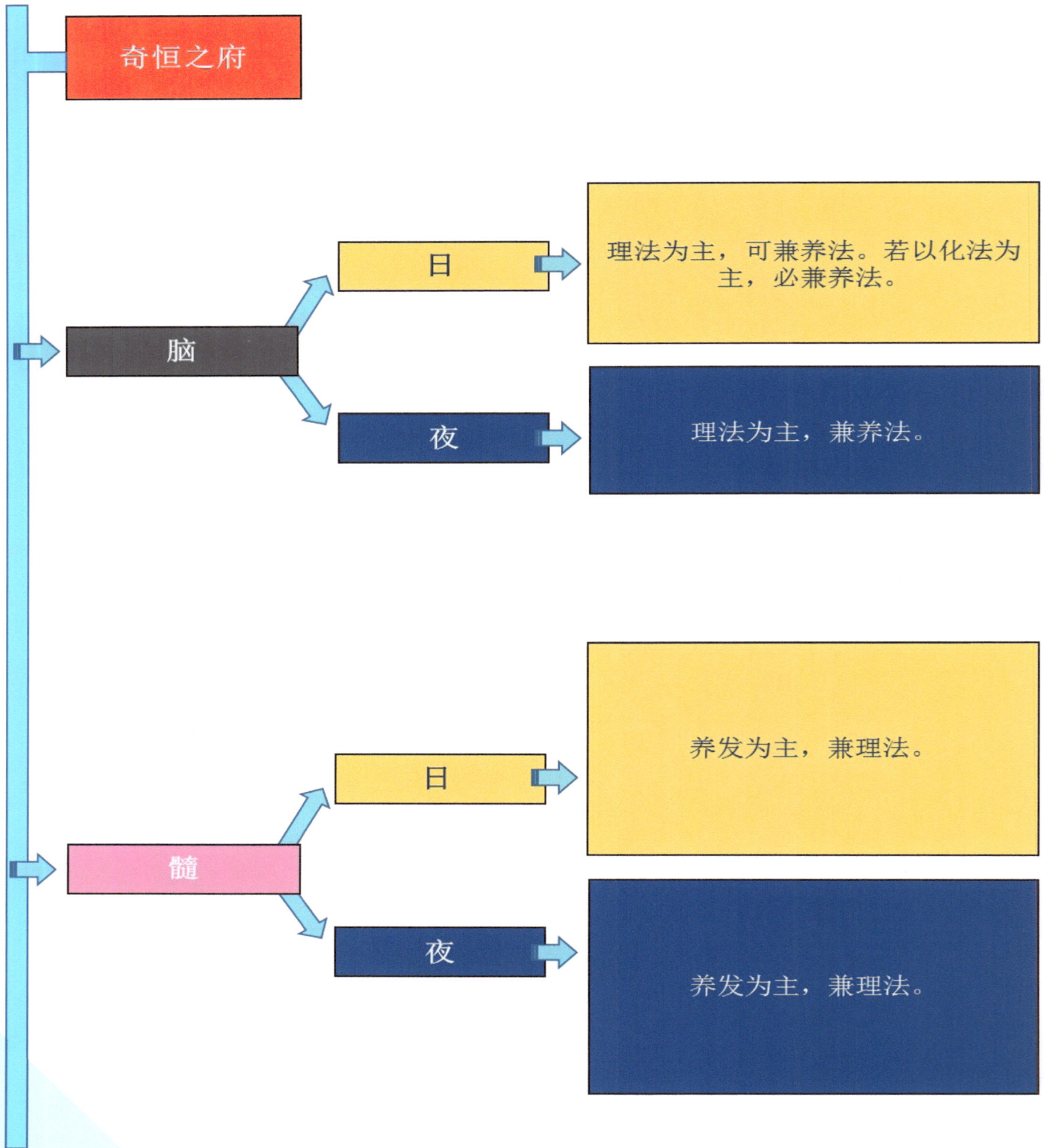

奇恒之府

脑

日 → 理法为主，可兼养法。若以化法为主，必兼养法。

夜 → 理法为主，兼养法。

髓

日 → 养发为主，兼理法。

夜 → 养发为主，兼理法。

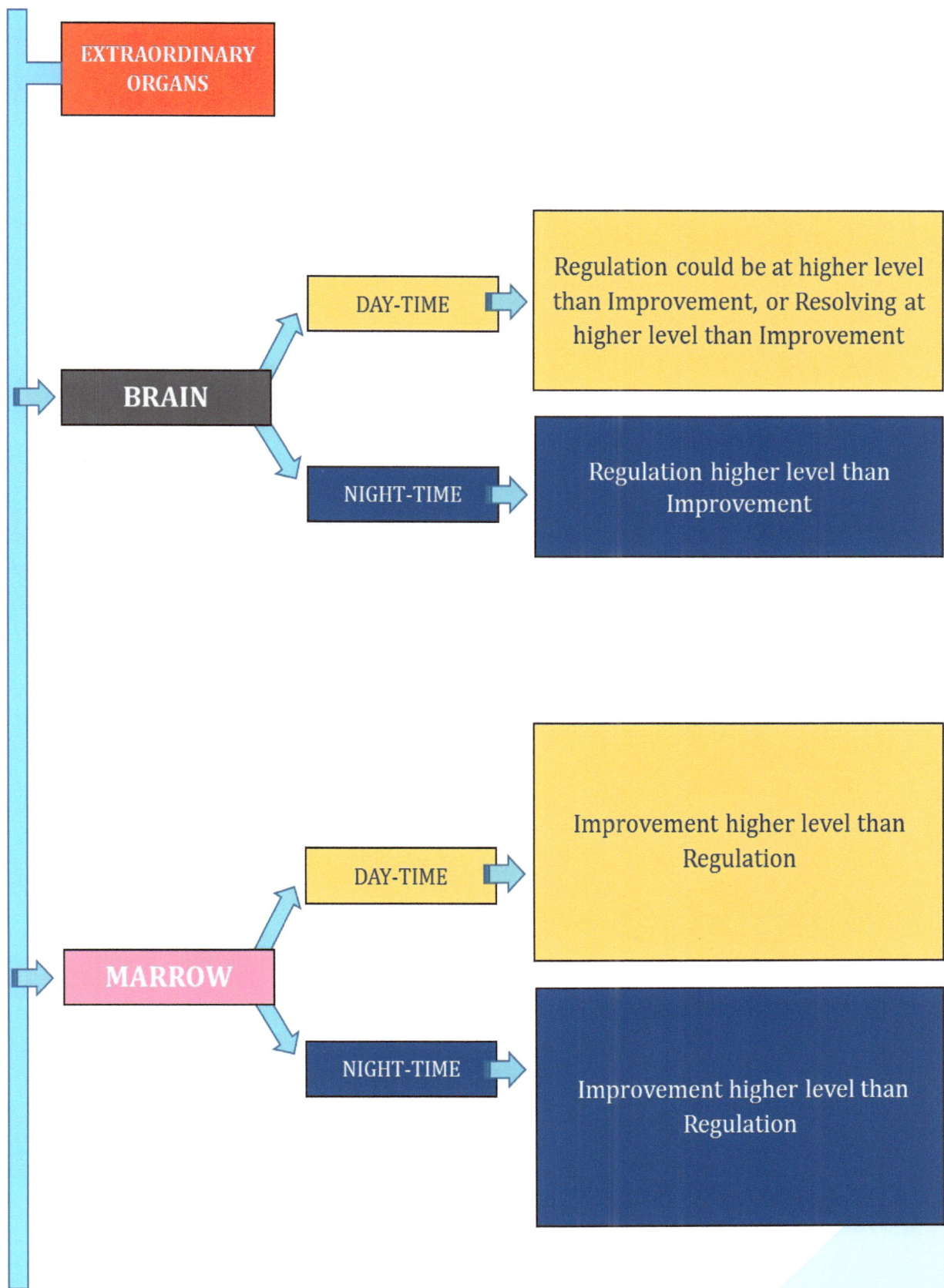

EXTRAORDINARY ORGANS

BRAIN

DAY-TIME → Regulation could be at higher level than Improvement, or Resolving at higher level than Improvement

NIGHT-TIME → Regulation higher level than Improvement

MARROW

DAY-TIME → Improvement higher level than Regulation

NIGHT-TIME → Improvement higher level than Regulation

95

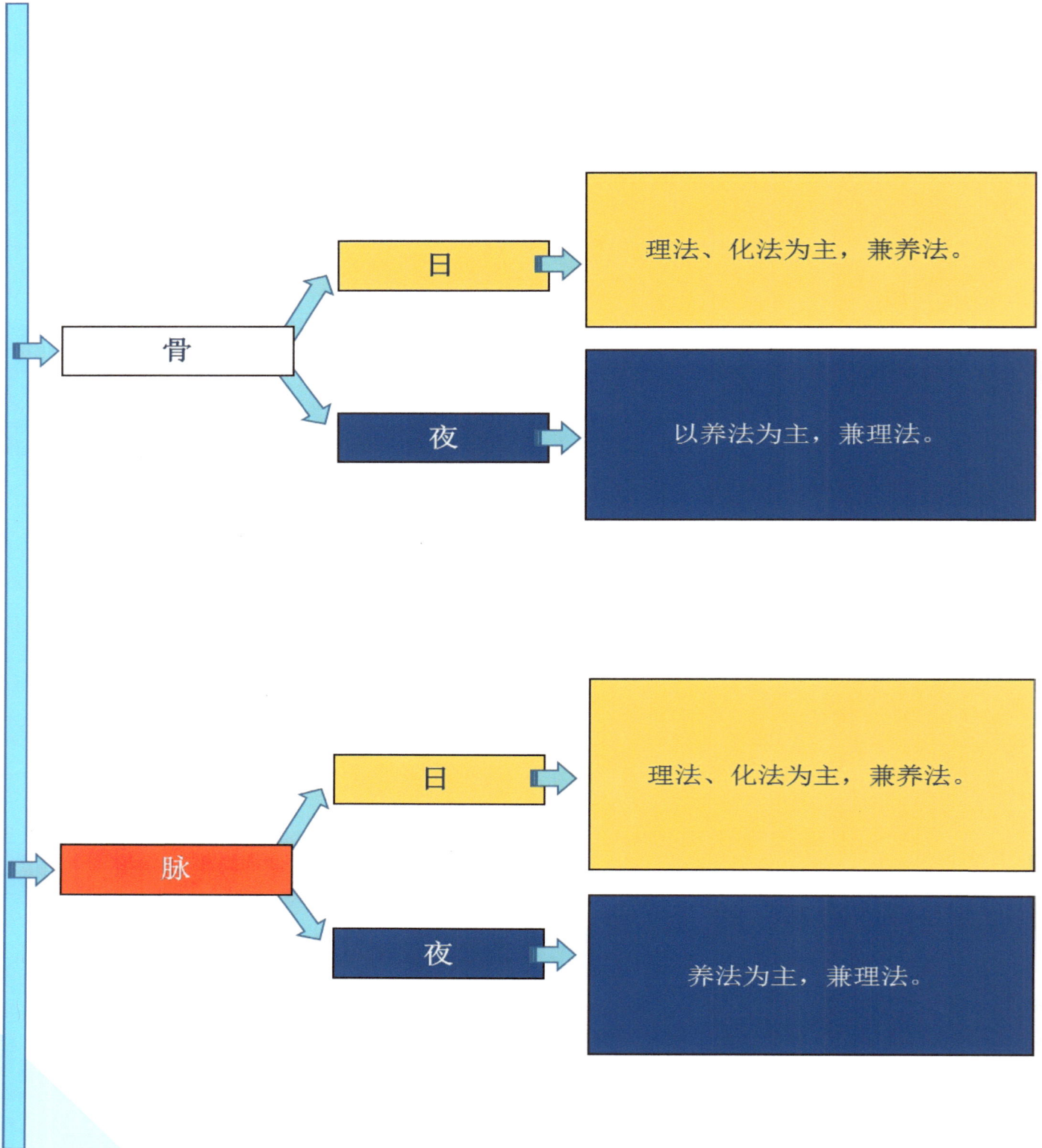

骨

日 → 理法、化法为主，兼养法。

夜 → 以养法为主，兼理法。

脉

日 → 理法、化法为主，兼养法。

夜 → 养法为主，兼理法。

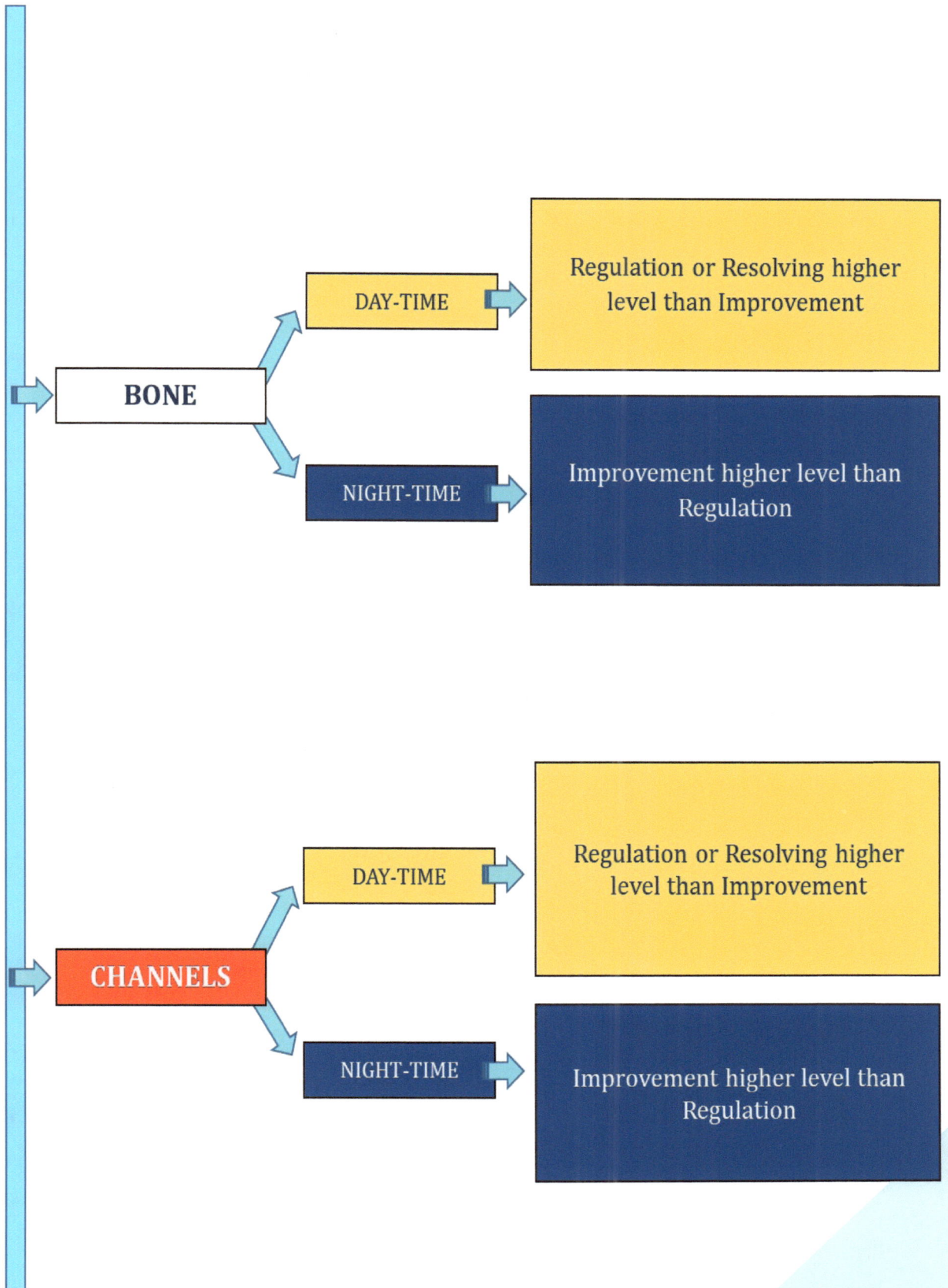

BONE

DAY-TIME → Regulation or Resolving higher level than Improvement

NIGHT-TIME → Improvement higher level than Regulation

CHANNELS

DAY-TIME → Regulation or Resolving higher level than Improvement

NIGHT-TIME → Improvement higher level than Regulation

97

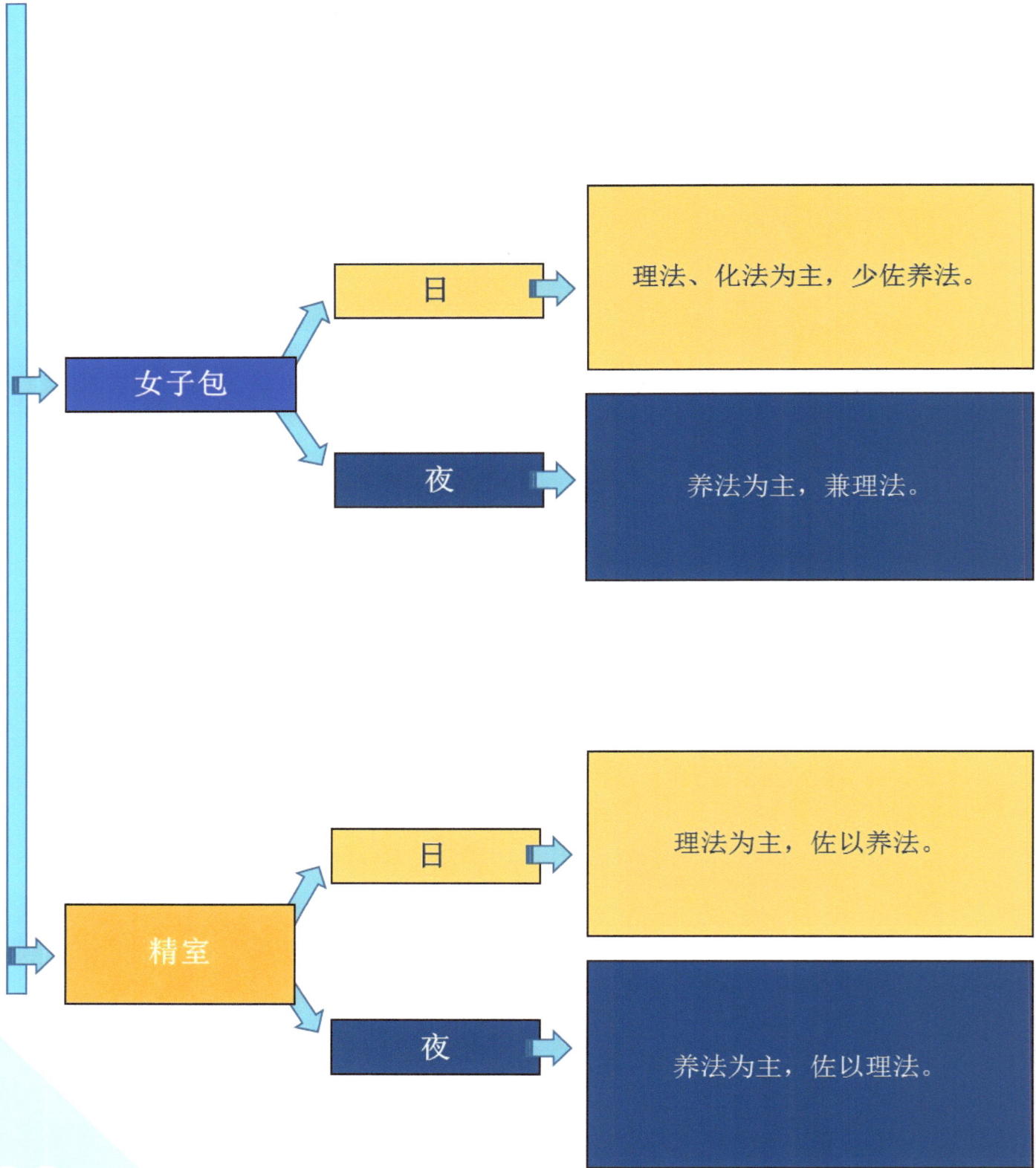

女子包

日 → 理法、化法为主，少佐养法。

夜 → 养法为主，兼理法。

精室

日 → 理法为主，佐以养法。

夜 → 养法为主，佐以理法。

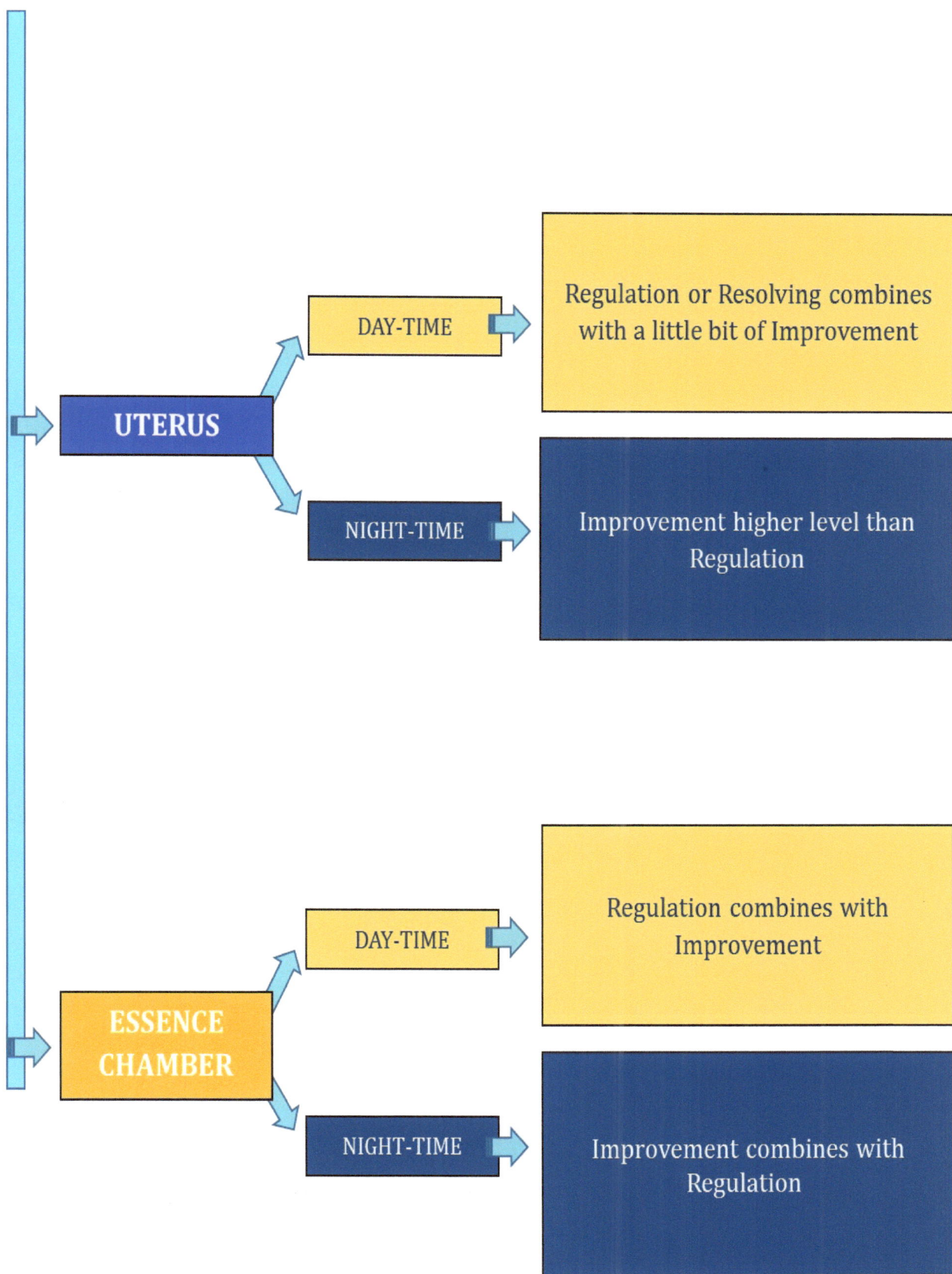

UTERUS

DAY-TIME → Regulation or Resolving combines with a little bit of Improvement

NIGHT-TIME → Improvement higher level than Regulation

ESSENCE CHAMBER

DAY-TIME → Regulation combines with Improvement

NIGHT-TIME → Improvement combines with Regulation

4.2.5 气血津液双极治则简述

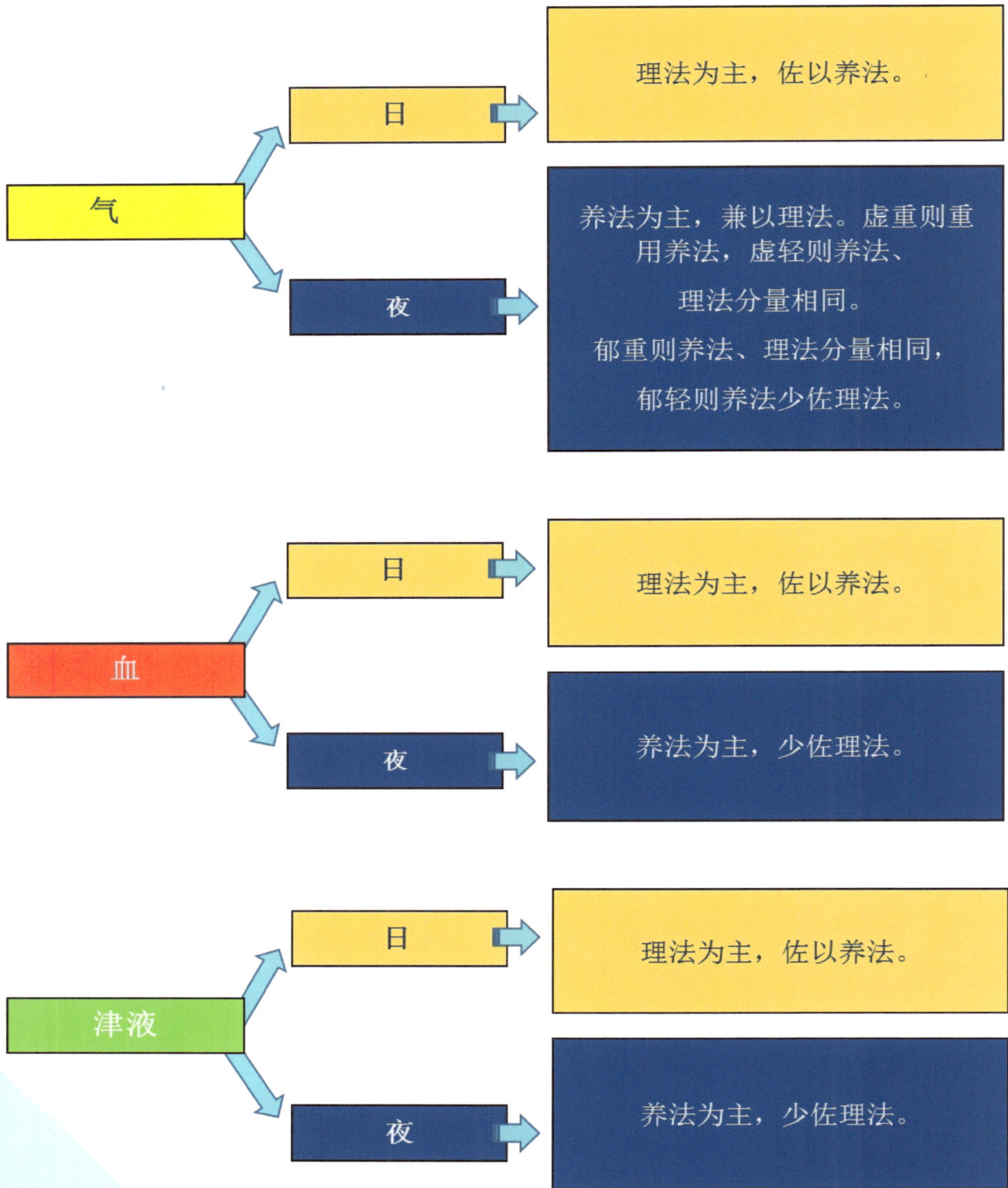

气

日 → 理法为主，佐以养法。

夜 → 养法为主，兼以理法。虚重则重用养法，虚轻则养法、
理法分量相同。
郁重则养法、理法分量相同，
郁轻则养法少佐理法。

血

日 → 理法为主，佐以养法。

夜 → 养法为主，少佐理法。

津液

日 → 理法为主，佐以养法。

夜 → 养法为主，少佐理法。

4.2.5. Brief Description of the Qi Blood and Body Fluid Therapeutic Principles of the Two Opposites

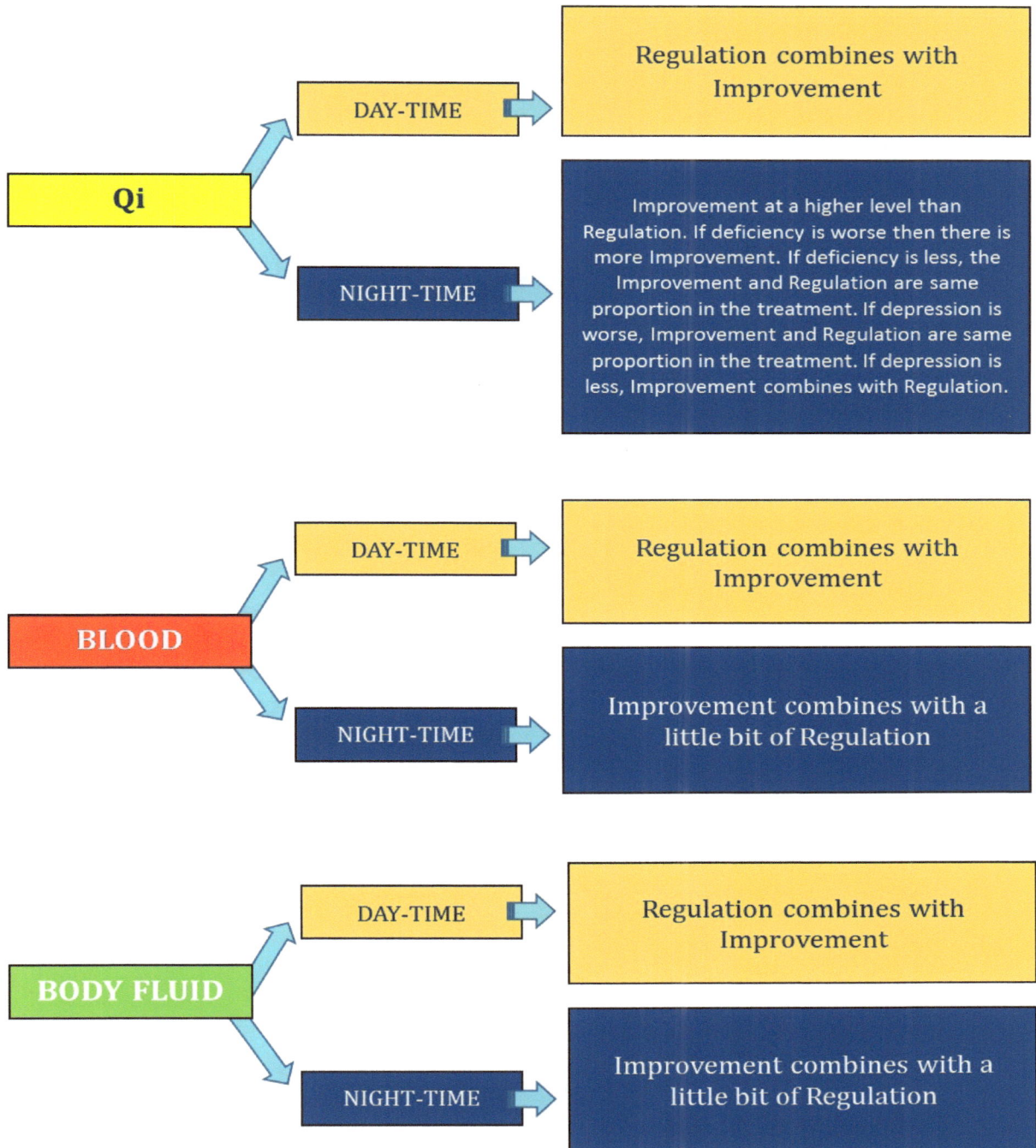

Qi

DAY-TIME → Regulation combines with Improvement

NIGHT-TIME → Improvement at a higher level than Regulation. If deficiency is worse then there is more Improvement. If deficiency is less, the Improvement and Regulation are same proportion in the treatment. If depression is worse, Improvement and Regulation are same proportion in the treatment. If depression is less, Improvement combines with Regulation.

BLOOD

DAY-TIME → Regulation combines with Improvement

NIGHT-TIME → Improvement combines with a little bit of Regulation

BODY FLUID

DAY-TIME → Regulation combines with Improvement

NIGHT-TIME → Improvement combines with a little bit of Regulation

5. 理论推演

双极理论的推演，首先是在阴阳的日夜相互转化规律基础上，确定双极理论的理论核心为阴阳双极。其次联系阴阳在脏腑五行、气血津液和经络腧穴中的运行规律，并结合脏腑五行、气血津液和经络腧穴在不同病理状态下的表现，逐个推演出它们各自的双极表现。再次将这一系列双极表现以阴阳为纲进行归类总结。最后以双极表现为指导，对现有中医治则进行总结，形成双极治则。

5. The Theoretical Deduction

The initial developmental inferences for the Two Opposites Theory, is derived from the day and night transformation rules of Yin and Yang which yield Yin and Yang Two Opposites is the theoretical core of the Two Opposites Theory. Combining the theoretical core along with the operational rules of; Zang Fu, Five Elements, Qi Blood and Body Fluid, Meridians and Points and the different performances of the pathological I was able to reason out the respective Manifestation of Two Opposites one by one. Further, based on Yin and Yang, I classified the series Manifestation of Two Opposites. Finally, being guided by the manifestation of two opposites, to summarize the existing therapeutic principles of Traditional Chinese Medicine and form the Therapeutic Principles of Two Opposites as presented.

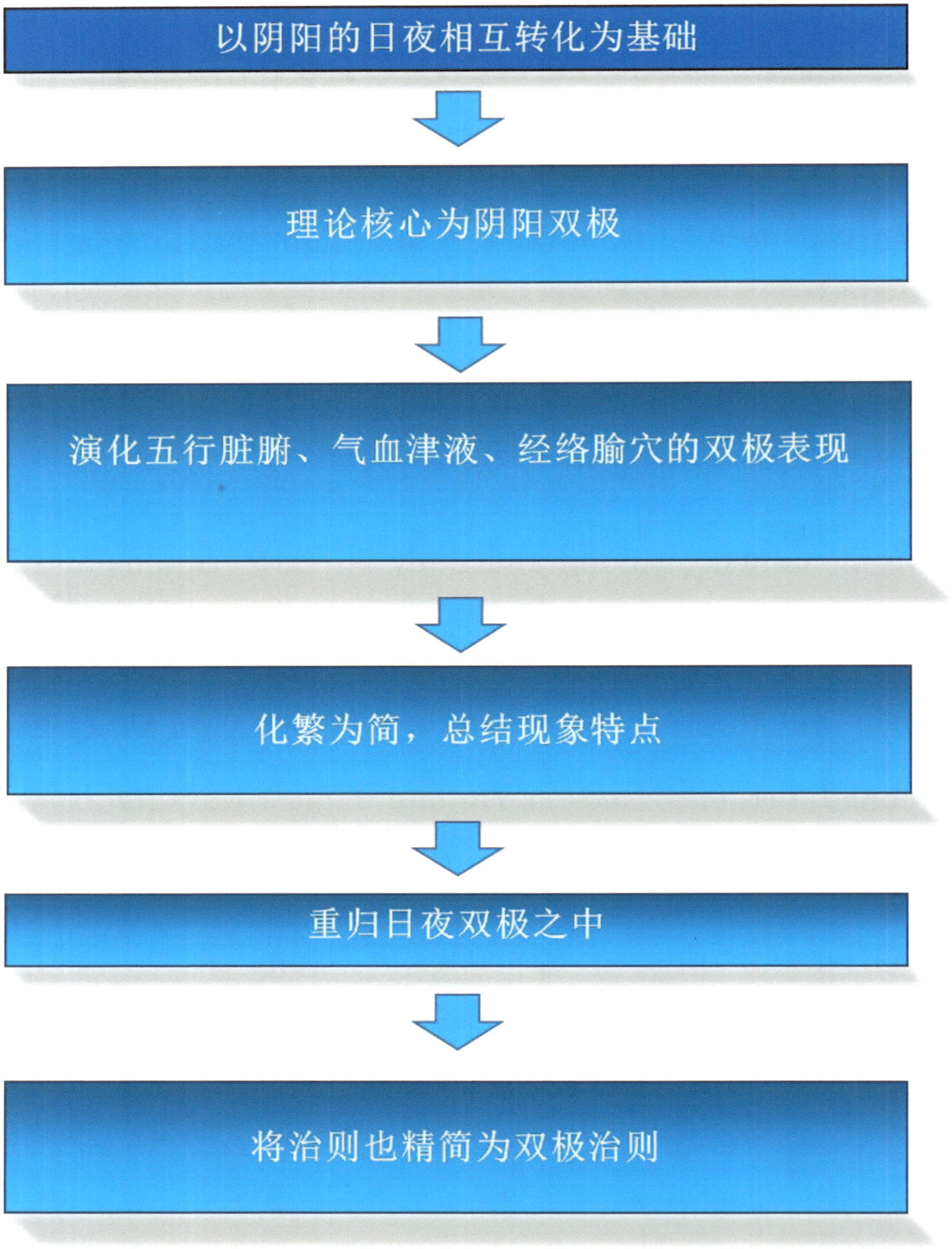

以阴阳的日夜相互转化为基础

↓

理论核心为阴阳双极

↓

演化五行脏腑、气血津液、经络腧穴的双极表现

↓

化繁为简，总结现象特点

↓

重归日夜双极之中

↓

将治则也精简为双极治则

Based on the transformation rules of Yin and Yang

⬇

Yin and Yang Two Opposites is the theoretical core of the Two Opposites Theory

⬇

Reason out the respective Manifestation of Two Opposites of Zang Fu and Five Elements, Qi Blood and Body Fluid, Meridians and Points

⬇

Change numerous for brief, summarize the manifestation characteristics

⬇

Return of day and night two opposites

⬇

Simplify the therapeutic principles to the Therapeutic Principles of Two Opposites

6. 理论思维导图

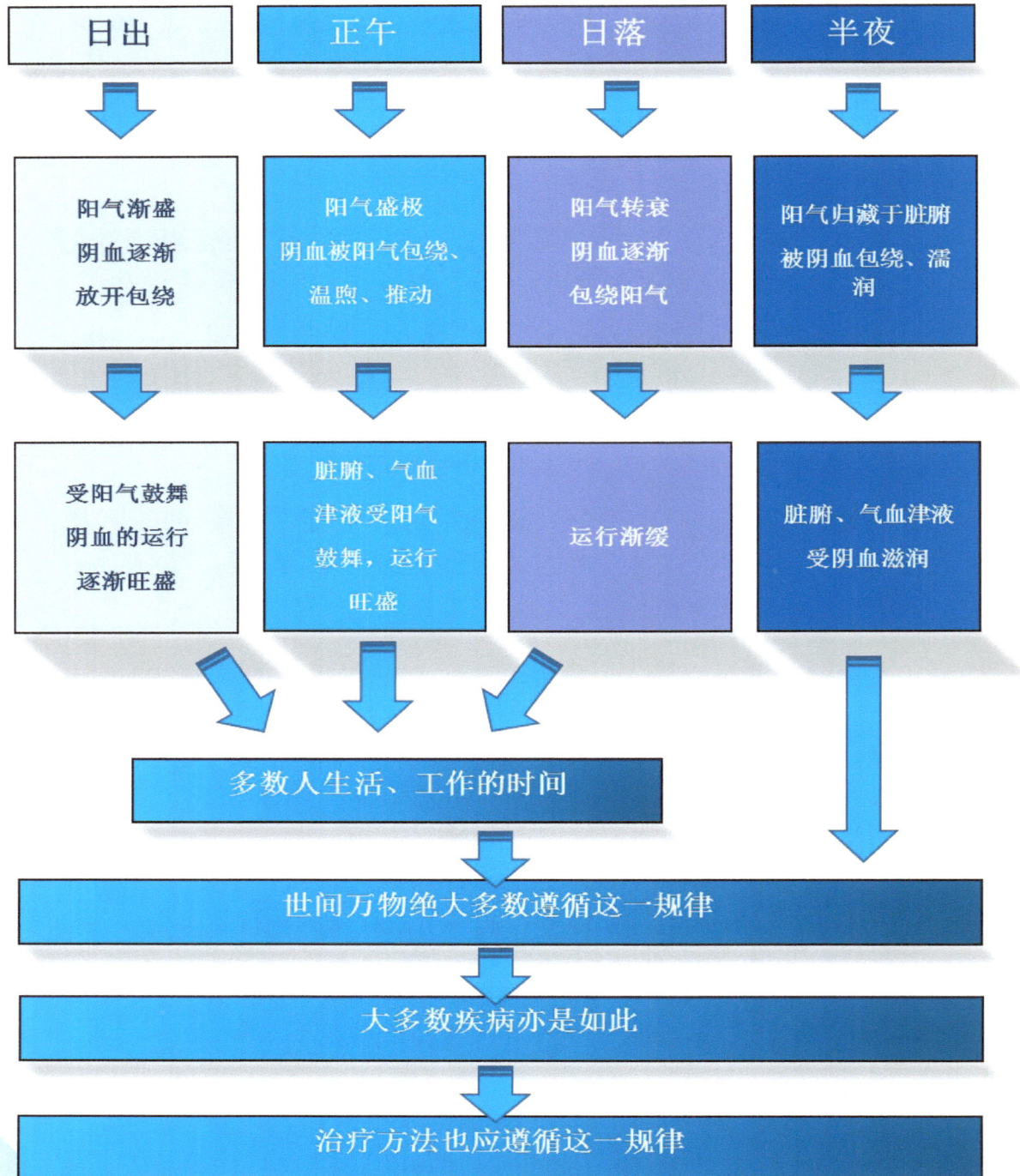

日出	正午	日落	半夜

↓ ↓ ↓ ↓

阳气渐盛 阴血逐渐 放开包绕	阳气盛极 阴血被阳气包绕、温煦、推动	阳气转衰 阴血逐渐 包绕阳气	阳气归藏于脏腑 被阴血包绕、濡润

↓ ↓ ↓ ↓

受阳气鼓舞 阴血的运行 逐渐旺盛	脏腑、气血 津液受阳气 鼓舞，运行 旺盛	运行渐缓	脏腑、气血津液 受阴血滋润

多数人生活、工作的时间

世间万物绝大多数遵循这一规律

大多数疾病亦是如此

治疗方法也应遵循这一规律

6. The Mind Map indicating the Reasoning of the Theory

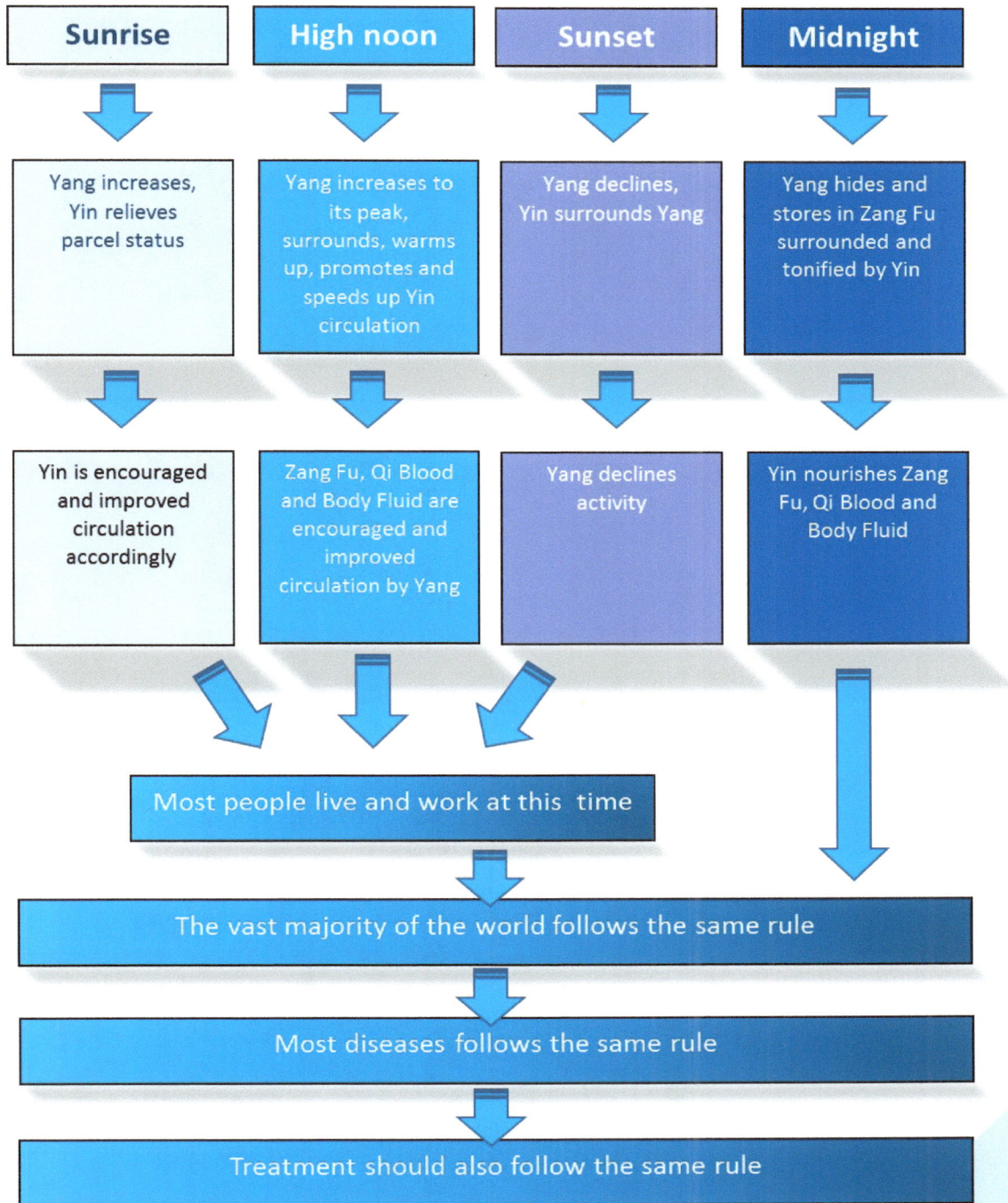

Sunrise	High noon	Sunset	Midnight

Yang increases, Yin relieves parcel status

Yang increases to its peak, surrounds, warms up, promotes and speeds up Yin circulation

Yang declines, Yin surrounds Yang

Yang hides and stores in Zang Fu surrounded and tonified by Yin

Yin is encouraged and improved circulation accordingly

Zang Fu, Qi Blood and Body Fluid are encouraged and improved circulation by Yang

Yang declines activity

Yin nourishes Zang Fu, Qi Blood and Body Fluid

Most people live and work at this time

The vast majority of the world follows the same rule

Most diseases follows the same rule

Treatment should also follow the same rule

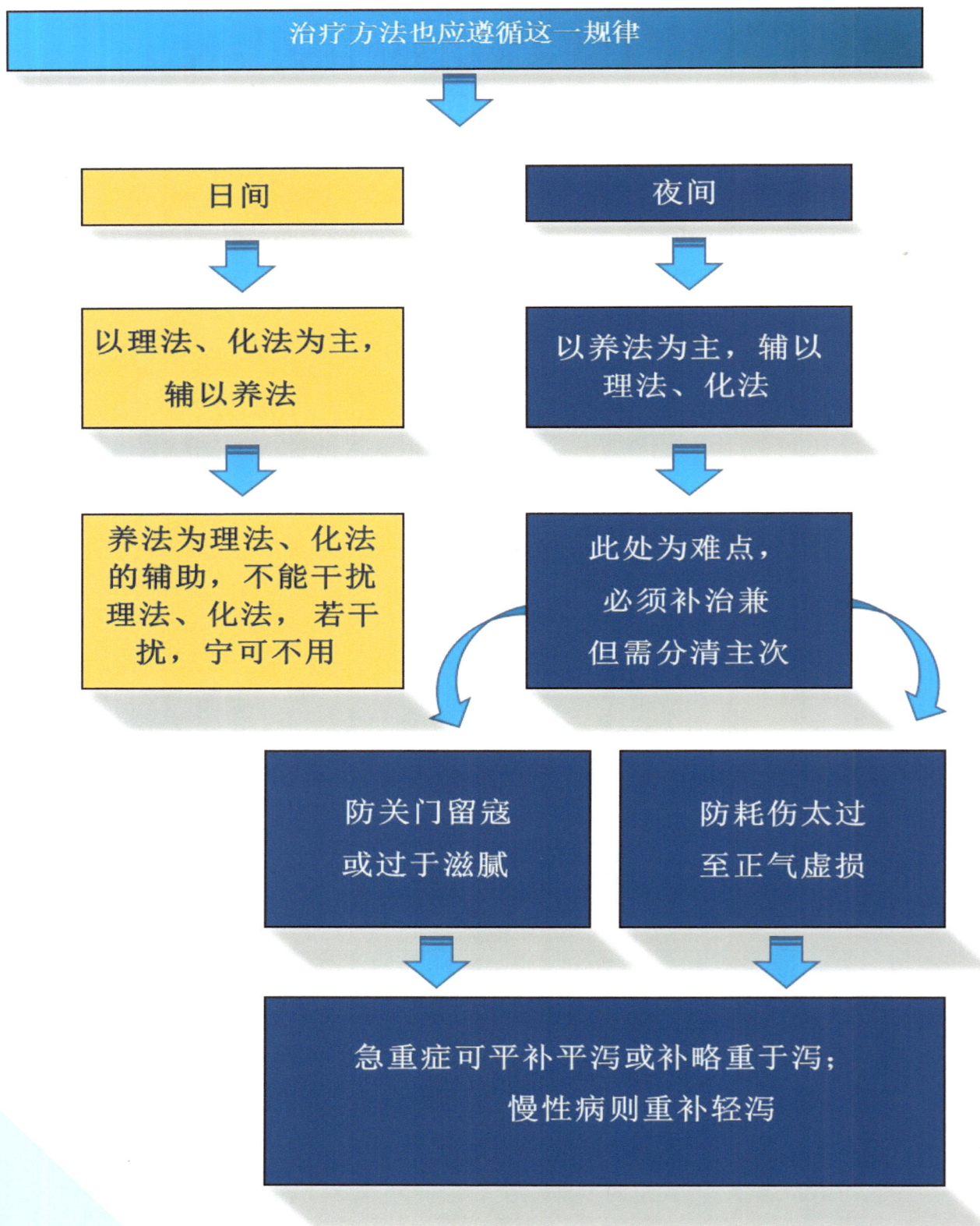

治疗方法也应遵循这一规律

日间	夜间
以理法、化法为主，辅以养法	以养法为主，辅以理法、化法
养法为理法、化法的辅助，不能干扰理法、化法，若干扰，宁可不用	此处为难点，必须补治兼但需分清主次

防关门留寇或过于滋腻

防耗伤太过至正气虚损

急重症可平补平泻或补略重于泻；慢性病则重补轻泻

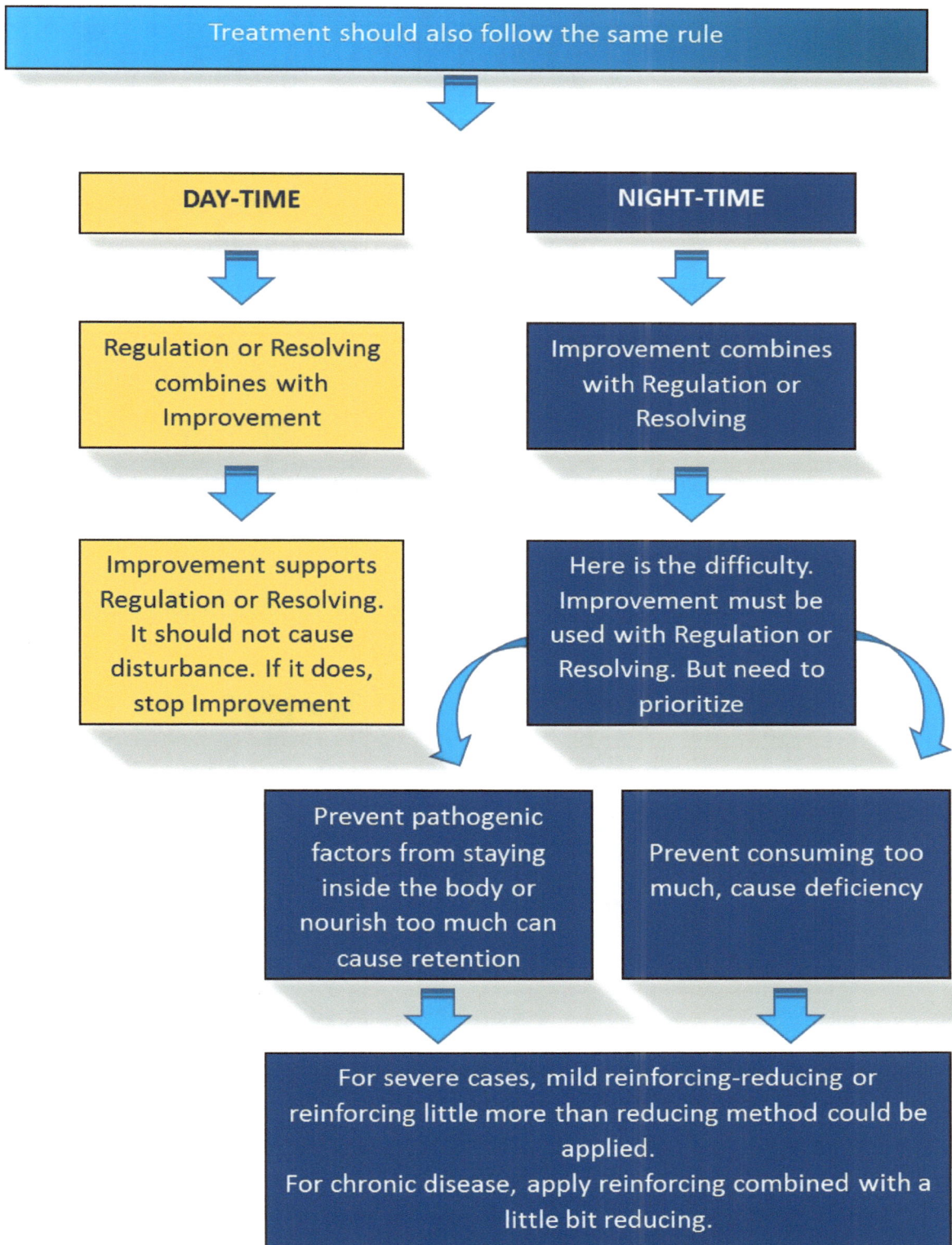

Treatment should also follow the same rule

DAY-TIME

NIGHT-TIME

Regulation or Resolving combines with Improvement

Improvement combines with Regulation or Resolving

Improvement supports Regulation or Resolving. It should not cause disturbance. If it does, stop Improvement

Here is the difficulty. Improvement must be used with Regulation or Resolving. But need to prioritize

Prevent pathogenic factors from staying inside the body or nourish too much can cause retention

Prevent consuming too much, cause deficiency

For severe cases, mild reinforcing-reducing or reinforcing little more than reducing method could be applied.
For chronic disease, apply reinforcing combined with a little bit reducing.

109

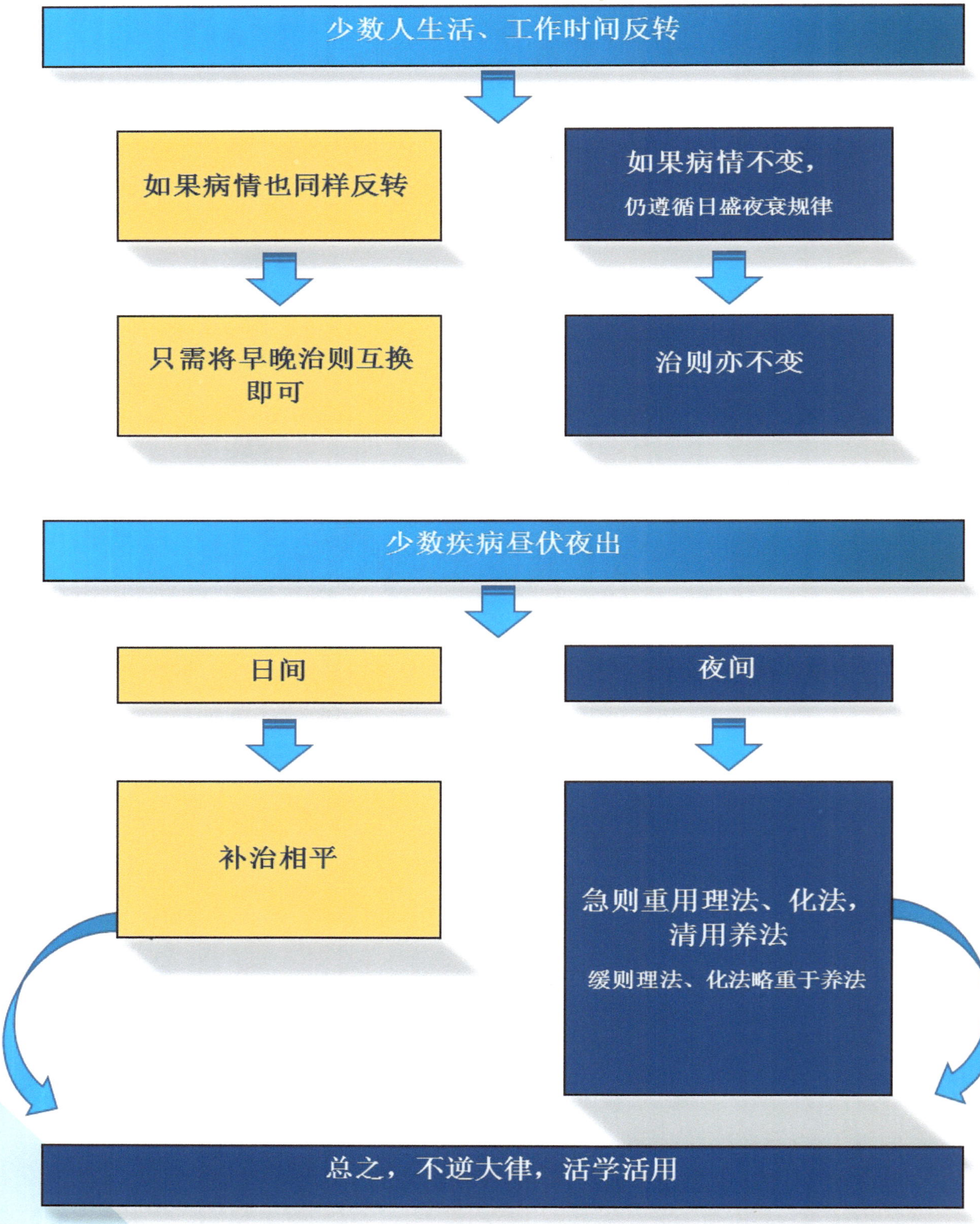

少数人生活、工作时间反转

如果病情也同样反转

只需将早晚治则互换即可

如果病情不变，
仍遵循日盛夜衰规律

治则亦不变

少数疾病昼伏夜出

日间

补治相平

夜间

急则重用理法、化法，
清用养法

缓则理法、化法略重于养法

总之，不逆大律，活学活用

110

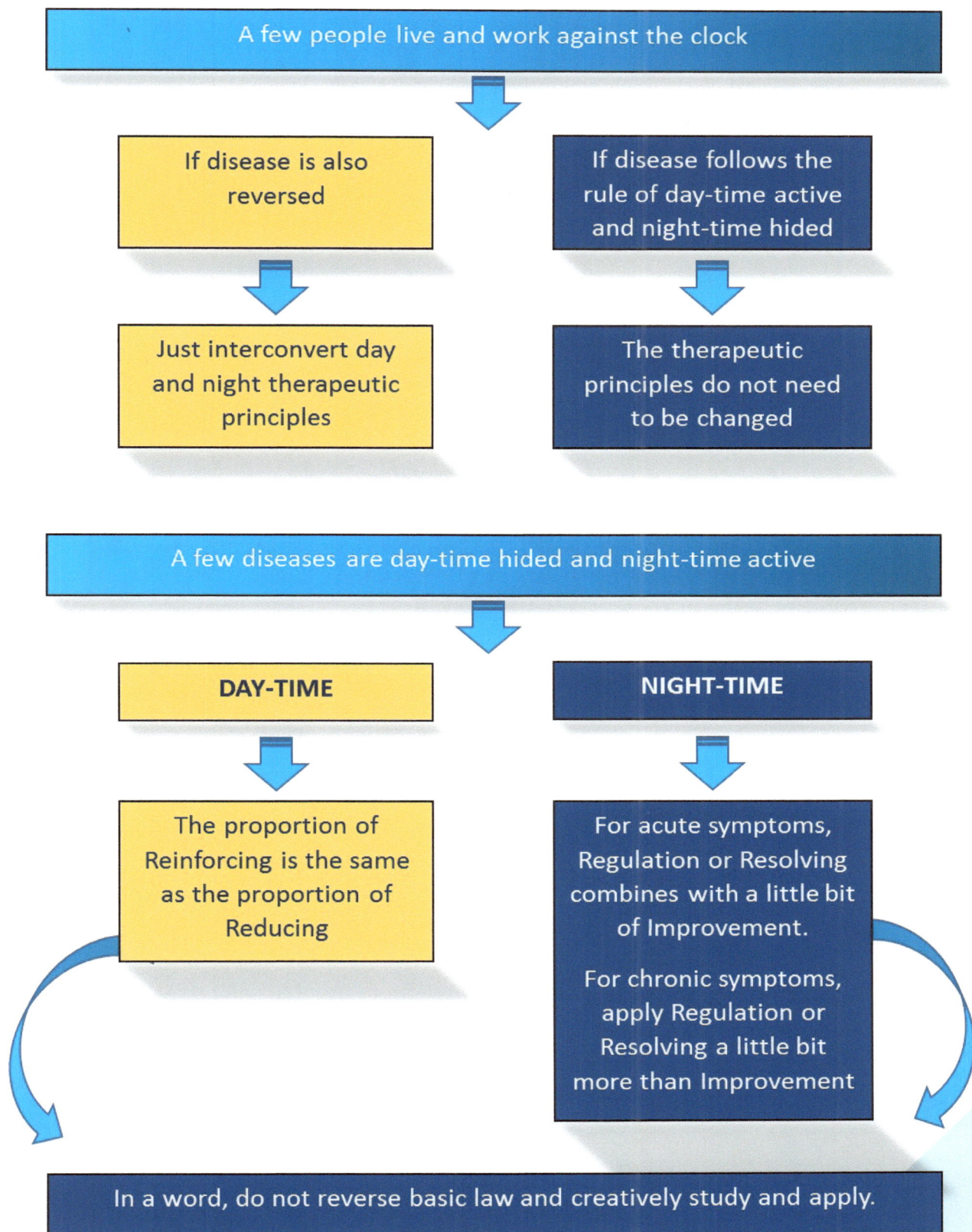

A few people live and work against the clock

If disease is also reversed

If disease follows the rule of day-time active and night-time hided

Just interconvert day and night therapeutic principles

The therapeutic principles do not need to be changed

A few diseases are day-time hided and night-time active

DAY-TIME

NIGHT-TIME

The proportion of Reinforcing is the same as the proportion of Reducing

For acute symptoms, Regulation or Resolving combines with a little bit of Improvement.

For chronic symptoms, apply Regulation or Resolving a little bit more than Improvement

In a word, do not reverse basic law and creatively study and apply.

7. 病例举证

7.1 病例1

病史：

男，20岁，二年前双手相继长出绿豆至豌豆大小的疣，呈圆形，表面粗糙，质地坚硬，新生疣呈淡粉色，成年疣为黄棕色。自汗。

7. Case Studies

7.1 Case 1

Information:

Male 20 years old. Two years ago large warts appeared on both of hands. They are as big as a mung bean or a pea. The warts were round in shaped, with rough and hard surfaces. The new born warts were light pink in color and the older warts were yellowish or brownish in color. The patient suffered from spontaneous sweating.

舌红有齿痕，苔淡黄滑腻。脉象，左手寸脉细数，关脉和尺脉细弱；右手寸脉浮取滑数，深按细弱，关脉滑，尺脉略沉。

辩证：

湿热蕴结上焦

His tongue body was red with teeth marks. The tongue coating was yellowish and greasy. The pulse palpation showed his left cun pulse was thin and rapid, the guan and chi pulses were thin and weak. The right hand pulses showed, the cun pulse was slippery and rapid on the superficial level but thin and weak on the deep level, his guan pulse was slippery and the chi pulse was slightly deep.

Pattern differentiation:

Damp heat accumulated in the Upper Jiao

治则：

日间——理法为主，佐以化法清上焦湿热；

夜间——养法为主，佐以理法养阴清热。

病因病机：

此病例呈现上焦湿热之邪泛溢于肌表之象，但与此同时又有阴血不足的症候。这是由于湿热蕴结日久，煎熬阴血所致。

Therapeutic principles:

Daytime:

Regulation combined with Resolving. Aim to drain and clear the Upper Jiao's damp-heat.

Nighttime:

Improvement combined with Regulation. Aim to nourish Yin and clear the heat.

Pathogen and Mechanism:

The symptoms presented within this case indicate the Upper Jiao's damp-heat has spilled over to the skin and muscles. Along with these symptoms this case also presents with symptoms of Yin and Blood deficiency. All these symptoms are caused by damp-heat that has been accumulating for a long time, resulting in the consumption of Yin and Blood of the whole body.

上午时分人体正气变得旺盛，湿热虽可为病，但由于正气的压制，难以发作。下午和傍晚时分正气渐衰，湿热之邪有机可乘，故多在此时趁势反扑。入夜之后，正气和湿热之邪均归于静谧，病势反而会见缓和。

In the morning, the function of Qi in the human body is to gather strength. Therefore, the damp-heat does not produce many symptoms in the morning because it is suppressed by the positive Qi in the body. Conversely in the afternoon and at dusk, the Qi in the body becomes weak. This provides an opportunity for the damp-heat to attack the human body. This is the exact reason why damp-heat symptoms worsen in the afternoon or at dusk. In the evening, both the positive Qi and the damp-heat of the human body go into hiding in the body in order to accumulate energy. This in turn makes the symptoms appear to be alleviated.

脾主运化，为驱除人体湿邪之要冲。而脾的生理功能在日夜之间是不同的。日间，脾之气血旺盛，运化之力最强。夜间，脾之阳气归藏，运化之力至弱，只能维持基本生理需要。因此，不管是从气血津液方面，还是脏腑方面上看，祛除湿之邪的最佳时机都在日间。

In the human body the spleen governs the transportation and transformation abilities, and it is the main organ involved in draining dampness out of the body. But the activities of the spleen are different between day and night. In the daytime, the Qi and Blood in the spleen are strong and sufficient. Therefore, allowing the transportation and transformation to function at its best. However, at night, the functions of transportation and transformation become weak due to the hiding of the spleen Yang. Their role is just to maintain the basic needs of the body. For these reasons, the best opportunity for treating dampness is in the daytime whether from the aspects of the Qi- Blood-Body Fluids or from the aspect of Zang-fu.

另一方面，阴血在日间是追随阳气的运动而动，并且接受阳气的温阳。而夜间则反过来滋养阳气，补充日间阳气的损耗。因此，夜间对阴血的补养，不仅能让阴血充足，还能间接供养阳气。

On the other hand, in the daytime, Yin and Blood follow the movement of Yang and Qi and are warmed by them. But at night, Yin and Blood in turn nourish Yang and Qi. Yin and Blood can replenish Yang and Qi consumed in the daytime during the night. Therefore, the nourishment of Yin and Blood at night not only can fill up Yin and Blood adequately, but also will tonify Yang and Qi indirectly.

　　所以在治则选取上，日间治则以理法和化法联合使用，目的是助人体正气清上焦湿热，力求尽去毒害。夜间治则以养法和理法联合使用，目的是养阴清热固护人体正气，同时兼清余毒。

Based on such analysis, when we choose the options of the therapeutic principles for this case, the daytime therapeutic principle is Regulation combined with Resolving aimed at draining the dampness, tonifying the spleen, and clearing away the pathogenic heat. This principle can help resolve the damp-heat in the Upper Jiao. The night therapeutic principle is Improvement combined with Regulation. Its aim is to benefit Yin and clear heat, while at the same time clearing the residual toxins.

处方：

日方：

天花粉 15 克

半夏 10 克

黄芩 5 克

陈皮 10 克

茯苓 10 克

蒲公英 10 克

紫花地丁 5 克

桔梗 5 克

白前 10 克

夜方：

白芍 5 克

黑芝麻 10 克

木香 5 克

生地黄 5 克

Prescription:

Daytime Formula:

Tian Hua Fen 15g

Ban Xia 10g

Huang Qin 5g

Chen Pi 10g

Fu Ling 10g

Pu Gong Ying 10g

Zi Hua Di Ding 5g

Jie Geng 5g

Bai Qian 10g

Nightime Formula:

Bai Shao 5g

Hei Zhi Ma 10g

Mu Xiang 5g

Sheng Di Huang 5g

服法说明：

上方 7 付，服用 7 天。饭后半小时服用。治疗期间，禁食生海鲜和水产品，禁食酒水，禁止吸烟。

后续治疗：

7 日后第一次复诊，无新生疣出现，已有的疣的数量减少超过 50%。无自汗。诊断后，原方继续服用。

14 日后第二次复诊，仅余 5 个已有的疣，并且有明显的萎缩消失迹象。舌尖略红。滑脉减轻。于是随证将前方改动后如下：

Directions:

7 days. Take each formula one and a half hours after a meal. Patient should not eat any kind of marine plants or animals nor should they drink alcohol or smoke during the entire treatment process.

Follow-up Treatment:

After 7days, during the first subsequent visit, if there are no newly born warts and the amount of adult warts were reduced over 50% and no spontaneous sweats were reported. The original formula will continue to be taken for another 7 days.

After 14 days, during the second subsequent visit, there were only 5 adult warts on the hands. There were signs of atrophy in the remaining 5 warts. The tip of the patient's tongue was a little red and a slippery pulse presented. So modifications were made to the original formula.

日方：

天花粉 10 克

半夏 5 克

黄芩 5 克

陈皮 5 克

茯苓 10 克

蒲公英 10 克

紫花地丁 5 克

桔梗 5 克

白前 10 克

夜方：

白芍 5 克

黑芝麻 10 克

木香 5 克

生地黄 5 克

酸枣仁 5 克

川芎 5 克

茯苓 5 克

Daytime Formula:

Tian Hua Fen 10g

Ban Xia 5g

Huang Qin 5g

Chen Pi 5g

Fu Ling 10g

Pu Gong Ying 10g

Zi Hua Di Ding 5g

Jie Geng 5g

Bai Qian 10g

Nighttime Formula:

Bai Shao 5g

Hei Zhi Ma 10g

Mu Xiang 5g

Sheng Di Huang 5g

Suan Zao Ren 5g

Chuan Xiong 5g

Fu Ling 5g

21 日后第三次复诊，仅余 2 个已有的疣，并且有明显的萎缩消失迹象。左手脉正常脉象；右手脉咯戴滑象。于是随证将前方改动后如下：

日方：

天花粉 10 克

半夏 10 克

黄芩 5 克

陈皮 10 克

茯苓 10 克

蒲公英 10 克

紫花地丁 5 克

桔梗 5 克

白前 10 克

白鲜皮 5 克

After 21 days, on the third subsequent visit, only 2 adult warts remained on the hands. There were obvious signs of atrophy in these 2 remaining warts. The patient's left hand pulse was normal. The right hand pulse was a little slippery. Further modifications were made to the prior formula.

Daytime Formula:

Tian Hua Fen 10g

Ban Xia 10g

Huang Qin 5g

Chen Pi 5g

Fu Ling 10g

Pu Gong Ying 10g

Zi Hua Di Ding 5g

Jie Geng 5g

Bai Qian 10g

Bai Xian Pi 5g

夜方：

白芍 5 克

阿胶 5 克

木香 5 克

生地黄 5 克

酸枣仁 5 克

川芎 5 克

茯苓 5 克

28 日后第四次复诊，双手无任何新生疣和成年疣。此后随访 2 周，仍无新生疣出现。患者治愈。

Nighttime Formula:

Bai Shao 5g

E Jiao 5g

Mu Xiang 5g

Sheng Di Huang 5g

Suan Zao Ren 5g

Chuan Xiong 5g

Fu Ling 5g

After 28 days, during the fourth subsequent visit, there were no newly born or adult warts present on the hands. This was followed by two more weeks of follow up checks on the patient. The results of his follow up showed no new warts. The patient was completely cured.

7.2 病例 2

病史：

男，34 岁，患者自述昨夜右侧耳尖直上靠近区巅顶域突发刺痛。睡觉后，疼痛加剧，时来时止，整夜未睡。现患者自觉头痛如针刺，时作时止。头痛发作时放射至整个右侧头部，向下放射至右耳及右侧牙齿，向前放射至右眼，导致疼痛发作时右眼无法睁开。同时今日晨起后右侧咽喉肿痛，做吞咽动作会使咽痛加剧，甚至引发头痛。患者自述头痛日间重于夜间。

7.2 Case 2

Information:

Male, 34 years old. Patient reports he suddenly felt stabbing pain the area from apex of right ear to vertex of the head yesterday evening. When he went to bed, the pain was aggravated then came and went. He was unable to sleep the entire night. Today, patient reports pain like needles and it comes and goes. The pain radiates to the whole right side of head and down to the right side ear and teeth then radiated to the front end of right eye. Patient was unable to open right eye due to pain. After this morning, patient felt right side throat was painful and swollen. Swallowing makes sore throat pain worse and caused a headache. Patient said that headache was worse in the daytime.

　　舌红有裂纹和齿痕，苔黄呈剥落苔。脉象，左手脉浮紧有力，尺脉深按虚弱无力；右手寸脉轻取浮紧有数象，重按无力，关脉轻取浮大而有力，重按无力，尺脉略弱。

Tongue was red with cracks and teeth marks. Tongue coating was peeled and yellow. The pulse palpation showed his left hand pulse was floating, tight and forceful but chi pulse was deep and weak. His right hand pulse was floating, tight and rapid on the superficial level, but weak on deep level. Guan pulse of right hand was floating big and forceful, but weak on deep level. Chi pulse was weaker.

辩证：

风寒袭表，入里化热，兼气阴两虚

治则：

日间——重用化法疏风解表，通经活络，清热消肿；

夜间——重用养法养阴蕴气，少配理法行气活血。

140

Pattern differentiation:

Wind cold invades and transforms to heat inside of body with Qi and Yin deficiency.

Therapeutic principles:

Daytime:

Use Resolving to dispel wind, relieve exterior, open channels, clearing and activating the channels and collaterals, clearing heat and diminishing swelling.

Nighttime:

Use Improvement to nourish Yin and tonify Qi combined with a little bit of Regulation to move Qi and Blood.

病因病机：

此病例呈现上焦为风寒所侵袭，致寒邪入里化热的症状，同时还有素体气阴两虚的症状。

日间阳气旺盛，正邪相争剧烈，所以头痛剧烈。同时由于阳气旺盛，此时用药助阳气攻邪更容易收到效果。所以日间重用化法，意在疏风解表，通经活络，清热消肿。

Pathogen and Mechanism:

The symptoms presented within this case indicate the Upper Jiao is invaded by wind cold and cold goes inside and transforms to heat while at the same time with Qi and Yin deficiency.

In the daytime, Yang is strong and active. The struggle between the vital energy and the pathogenic factor is fierce. That causes the headache to be worse and aggravated. Meanwhile, because Yang is strong and active using herbs to support Yang is easy to attack pathogenic factor and obtain a good result. Therefore, using Resolving is aimed at dispelling wind, relieving exterior, opening channels, clearing and activating the channels and collaterals, clearing heat and diminishing swelling.

夜间阳气潜伏，阴血阳气润养于内。但由于阴血不足，阳气得不到足够的蕴养，不能彻底祛邪于外。所以夜间以养法为主，意在养阴蕴气，少佐理法行气活血。

144

In the nighttime, Yang goes into hiding. Yin and Yang are nourished inside of human body. But because Yin is deficient, Yang cannot get enough nourishment from Yin. It cannot dispel pathogenic factors outside totally. Therefore, using Improvement is aimed at nourishing Yin and tonifying Qi combined with a little bit Regulation to move Qi and Blood.

处方：

日方：

川芎 30 克

白芷 30 克

羌活 30 克

细辛 20 克

葛根 10 克

地龙 10 克

天花粉 15 克

黄芩 15 克

紫花地丁 15 克

薄荷 30 克

Prescription:

Daytime Formula:

Chuan Xiong 30g

Bai Zhi 30g

Qiang Huo 30g

Xi Xin 20g

Ge Gen 10g

Di Long 10g

Tian Hua Fen 15g

Huang Qin 15g

Zi Hua Di Ding 15g

Bo He 30g

夜方：

紫河车 10 克

龟板 10 克

鹿角霜 5 克

锁阳 5 克

淫羊藿 15 克

山药 10 克

地龙 10 克

牛膝 5 克

补骨脂 5 克

当归 10 克

阿胶 10 克

远志 5 克

百合 5 克

郁金 5 克

香附 10 克

麦冬 5 克

沙参 5 克

Nighttime Formula:

Zi He Che 10g

Gui Ban 10g

Lu Jiao Shuang 5g

Suo Yang 5g

Yin Yang Huo 15g

Shan Yao 10g

Di Long 10g

Niu Xi 5g

Bu Gu Zhi 5g

Dang Gui 10g

A Jiao 10g

Yuan Zhi 5g

Bai He 5g

Yu Jin 5g

Xiang Fu 10g

Mai Dong 5g

Sha Shen 5g

服法说明：

上方 7 付，服用 7 天。饭前半小时服用。治疗期间，禁食生海鲜和水产品，禁食辛辣、酒水，禁止吸烟。

结果：

当日服用日方后 2 小时，头痛明显缓解。服用夜方后，夜间头痛未发作，睡眠恢复正常。服用三日后，头痛时有发作，疼痛程度减轻。7 日后复诊，虽然仍时而头痛，但程度很轻，并且头痛位置固定不移。咽喉肿痛消失。于是将日方组成不变，用量减半，夜方不变，继续服用一周。5 日后，患者反馈，头痛消失。于是嘱患者停用日方，服完夜方即可。

Directions:

7 days. Take each formula one and a half hours before a meal. Patient should not eat any kind of marine plants or animals nor should they eat spicy food, drink alcohol or smoke during the entire treatment process.

Result:

2 hours after taking daytime formula, headache relieved. Headache did not return at night after taking the nighttime formula. Sleep returned to normal. After taking the formula three days, headache returned sometimes but pain relieved. After 28 days, during the subsequent visit, although sometimes still has a headache, it is very light and never radiating. The sore throat disappeared. The constitution of daytime formula was not change, but dosage was decreased by half. The nighttime formula did not change. These formulas were continued for another week. After 5 days, feedback of patient was headache disappeared. Therefore, patient was advised to discontinued daytime formula but to complete taking the nighttime formula as previously directed.

7.3 病例 3

病史：

男，63 岁，高血压病史多年，晨起血压升高，头晕目眩，情志抑郁，夜寐不安，时有惊醒，夜尿多而不净，尿色黯黄，口干。

舌尖边红，苔黄厚腻，左手脉弦，右手脉革。

辩证：

血虚生风，心肾不交

7.3 Case 3

Information:

Male, 63 years old. He had suffered from hypertension for years. His blood pressure was typically higher in the morning and felt dizziness and depression. At night, he had interrupted sleep by awakening many times with frequent dripping urination. The urine was dark yellow in color and his mouth was dry.

The tip and sides of the tongue were red with a yellow thick greasy coating. The pulse palpation showed his left pulse was wiry, whereas his right pulse was leathery.

Pattern differentiation:

Internal wind caused by blood deficiency with poor interactions between heart and kidneys.

治则：

日间——理法为主意在疏肝理气，佐以养法、化法意在健脾化痰；

夜间——理法、化法合用与养法相平，意在潜阳熄风，养血安神。

154

Therapeutic principles:

Daytime:

Regulation focused on soothing and regulating liver Qi. Combined with Improvement to tonify spleen and Resolving to drain dampness.

Nighttime:

Regulation is at a higher level than Resolving while both are in same proportion as Improvement. Adopt the combined therapeutic methods with the purpose of suppressing the Yang to quench wind and nourish the blood to tranquilize the mind.

病因病机：

此病例呈现虚风内动的征象。血虚，日间会出现气无所依的表现。表现在肝的阴血不足上，就会出现血虚，肝气无以依靠，扰动一身之气，形成内风的表现。而晨起之时正是一天中阳气复苏，逐步增强的时刻。此时，阳气若没有阴血的依靠，很容易升发太过，导致病人晨起血压过高，头晕目眩。肝气扰动，心神不宁。若肝气扰动而导致气机郁滞，则会出现情志抑郁不疏。

Pathogen and Mechanism:

This case shows the symptoms of internal wind deficiency. In the daytime, Qi would lose dependence on anything inside the body. When liver Yin and Blood are deficient, there is nothing liver Qi can depend on and that would disturb the Qi of the whole body, thus causing the internal wind symptoms. When we wake up in the morning, Yang Qi starts to revive and enhance gradually. At this time, if Qi loses dependence upon Yin and Blood, it will ascend too fast, and that would result in the morning high blood pressure and dizziness of the patient. If liver Qi bothers or disturbs the heart, the patient will suffer from anxiety and restlessness. And if liver Qi disturbs, the patient might suffer from Qi stagnation, feeling emotionally depressed.

血虚日久，必然导致阴虚，累及心肾。可导致心肾不交，则会出现夜间多梦难寐，夜尿频数。阴血不足，虚火上扰，则出现口干，尿黄等症状。

所以，在治则的选用上，日间以疏理肝气，健脾化痰为主要思想。而夜间则要在补养阴血的同时，疏理肝气，防次日清阳之气升发太过。

When blood deficiency lasts for a long time, it will cause Yin deficiency and would therefore influence heart and kidneys. That may cause failure in the interactions of heart and kidneys, showing symptoms such as dreaminess, insomnia and frequent urination at night. If Yin Blood is deficient, the pathogenic deficiency fire will go up with disturbances, thus showing symptoms such as dry mouth and yellow-color urine.

Therefore, the selection of therapeutic principles for the daytime should be focused on the soothing and regulation of liver Qi, strengthening of spleen functions as well as the resolution of dampness. But, night therapeutic principle is aimed at nourishing Yin and Blood accompanied by the soothing of liver Qi to avoid the rapid ascending of the Yang in the next morning.

此病例的治法，是顺应疾病的发病规律而治。本病的发展规律实际上是始发于夜间，发作于日间。所以，在制定治则时夜间治则的制定尤为重要。

The therapeutic method of this case is based on the compliance with the law of the occurrences and development of the diseases. The law of the development of this case indicates that the disease originated at night but became active and obvious in the daytime. Therefore, it is especially important to work out the therapeutic principles for the night treatment when making plans for the treatment of all diseases.

处方：

日方：

柴胡 10 克

香附 10 克

阿胶 5 克

石决明 5 克

牛膝 5 克

山药 5 克

茯苓 10 克

半夏 5 克

陈皮 5 克

Prescription:

Daytime Formula:

Chai Hu 10g

Xiang Fu 10g

E Jiao 5g

Shi Jue Ming 5g

Niu Xi 5g

Shan Yao 5g

Fu Ling 10g

Ban Xia 5g

Chen Pi 5g

夜方：

柴胡 5 克

香附 5 克

阿胶 10 克

熟地 10 克

石决明 5 克

天麻 5 克

龙骨 5 克

酸枣仁 10 克

合欢皮 10 克

服法说明：

上方 7 付，服用 7 天。饭后半小时服用。治疗期间，禁食酒水，禁止吸烟。

Nighttime Formula:

Chai Hu 5g

Xiang Fu 5g

E Jiao 10g

Shu Di 10g

Shi Jue Ming 5g

Tian Ma 5g

Long Gu 5g

Suan Zao Ren 10g

He Huan Pi 10g

Directions:

Use the formula for 7 days. Take every formula at half hour after meals. Any alcoholic drinks or smoking are forbidden during the entire treatment process.

结果：

当夜服用后，夜尿次数减少，睡眠质量明显改善，次日晨起，晕眩感减轻，情绪开朗。自测血压，血压正常。

Result:

The frequency of urination at night reduced in the first night, after using the formula. Sleeping quality improved significantly. The next day morning, dizziness was alleviated and his mood was cheerful. Patient checked blood pressure by himself and the result of blood pressure was normal. After one week, the patient's situation remained stable.

7.4 病例 4

病史：

女，25 岁，月经淋漓不止 3 个月。面色㿠白，皮肤干燥，倦怠乏力，纳差便溏，盗汗多梦，血色淡红，量多，四肢寒冷。

舌胖大有齿痕，苔薄白，左寸脉、关脉革，尺脉沉弱，右寸脉、关脉革，尺脉弱。

辩证：

气血两亏，气不摄血

7.4 Case 4

Information:

Female, 25 years old, metrostaxis 3 months. Patient presents with pale face, dry skin, and fatigue. She has no appetite and her digestion was poor with diarrhea. She dreams a lot combined with night sweats. Her menstrual color is light red and copious. She always feels her four limbs are cold.

Her tongue is swollen with teeth marks. The tongue coating is thin and white. Her left side cun and guan pulses are leathery. The chi pulse is deep and weak. Her right side cun and guan pulses are leathery also. The chi pulse is weak.

Pattern differentiation:

Qi and Blood deficiency, Qi cannot hold Blood.

治则：

日间——重用化法止血止亏；

夜间——重用养法养阴补血壮阳，少佐理法行气活血。

Therapeutic principles:

Daytime:

Use Resolving to stop bleeding and depleting.

Nighttime:

Use Improvement to nourish Yin and blood, tonify Yang and combine with a little bit Regulation to move Qi and Blood.

病因病机：

此病例呈现气血亏虚导致气不摄血的征象。该患者由于气虚，致使日间阳气无法有效推动血液运行，导致经脉、脏腑无法得到足够的充养，所以出现疲劳乏力，食欲减退，四肢寒冷等一系列的气血虚弱症状。由于血液的运行依赖气机的统摄才能在经脉内正常的流行。失去或缺乏气机的统摄，血液将无法正常在经脉内流行，进而出现血瘀或出血症状。日间由于人类活动增加导致血液流行速度较快，血液在得不到气的有效统摄下，血瘀或者出血症状相较于夜间会加重。而血瘀或出血的加重会进一步加重气虚的程度，造成恶性循环。这就是为什么，该患者会出现月经淋漓不止。

Pathogen and Mechanism:

This case shows the symptoms of Qi and Blood deficiency. This causes the Qi to be unable to hold Blood. Because patient has Qi deficiency, Qi cannot push Blood efficiently in the daytime. This results in the Meridians and Zang Fu loosing nourishment and showing a series Qi and Blood deficiency symptoms such as fatigue, decreased appetite and coldness in the four limbs. The movement of Blood in the meridians depends on the domination of Qi. Lost or lack of the domination of Qi, the Blood cannot float normally in the meridians. It will cause blood stasis or bleeding symptoms. In the daytime, due to human activities increase the speed of blood movement, blood stasis and bleeding are aggravated without the domination of Qi. Blood stasis and bleeding are also aggravated by the degree of the Qi deficiency. This causes a vicious cycle. Therefore, patient showed metrostaxis.

所以本病的日间治则应以化法为主，意在止血，打破恶性循环，停止身体内的恶性消耗。给夜间的补益气血打下基础。

血虚日久，阴液必然亏虚。阴血两虚，夜间阳气没有足够的阴血包绕，扰动心神，会出现多梦的症状。同样由于阳气失去阴血的包绕，不自主向身体外发散，导致体液随之散失，形成盗汗。

So the daytime therapeutic principle of this case is Resolving which aims to stop bleeding and malignant consumption and to destroy the vicious cycle. It can build a good foundation on reinforcing Qi and Blood in the nighttime.

Blood deficiency for a long time will cause Yin deficiency. Yin and Blood deficiency during the night will cause a lack of Yin and Blood needed to surround Yang. Yang will then bother heart spirit causing a lot of dreams. In the same way, losing Yin and Blood surrounding, Yang spreads out of human body involuntarily. Body fluid follows, Yang spreads outside and causes night sweats.

因此，夜间治则必须以养法为主，养血温经，滋养阳气，达到壮阳的效果。但是滋养过度，会导致滋腻碍胃、阻滞经脉等症候。所以在重用养法的同时，少佐以理法行气活血，既可以防患于未然，又可以加速滋养一身之气血阴液，一举两得。

夜间的补养和调理还可以为身体日间的固摄止血提供更多的能量，促使身体机制重建良性循环，对于治疗疾病起到积极促进作用。

Therefore, nighttime therapeutic principle must use Improvement aimed at nourishing blood, warming Meridians and tonifing Yang. Take caution reinforcing too much will cause stomach obstruction and meridians to be blocked. For this reason, combine a little bit Regulation to move Qi and Blood when using Improvement. This is not only nipping obstruction in the bud but also speeds up reinforcing Qi Blood and Body Fluid in the body. This will kill two birds with one stone.

In addition, using Improvement and Regulation in the nighttime can support more energy to dominate Blood and stop bleeding in the daytime. This prompts the body mechanism to rebuild a virtuous cycle and play a positive role for treating diseases.

处方：

日方：

血余碳 5 克

夜方：

熟地 15 克

白芍 15 克

当归 15 克

川芎 10 克

艾叶 10 克

香附 5 克

山药 10 克

茯苓 10 克

桂枝 5 克

五味子 10 克

178

Prescription:

Daytime Formula:

Xue Yu Tan 5g

Night Formula:

Shu Di 15g

Bai Shao 15g

Dang Gui 15g

Chuan Xiong 10g

Ai Ye 10g

Xiang Fu 5g

Shan Yao 10g

Fu Ling 10g

Gui Zhi 5g

Wu Wei Zi 10g

服法说明：

上方 7 付，服用 7 天。饭前半小时服用。治疗期间，禁食生海鲜和水产品，禁食辛辣、酒水，禁止吸烟。

结果：

次日患者服用日方后 2 小时左右，流血停止。夜方服用后当日盗汗减少，梦少。此后血止，3、4 日后盗汗消失，偶尔有梦。面色略见红润，体力逐渐恢复。于是 7 日后复诊，停用日方，继续服用夜方两周，病痊愈。

Directions:

7 days. Take each formula one and a half hours before a meal. Patient should not eat any kind of marine plants or animals nor should they eat spicy food, drink alcohol or smoke during the entire treatment process.

Result:

Bleeding stopped 2 hours after patient took the daytime formula. The same day patient had less dreams and night sweats after taking the nighttime formula. After she finished first day formula, the metrostaxis disappeared. In the third and fourth days, patient dreamed sometimes but had no night sweats. Her face is slight pink and she felt more energy. After 7days during the subsequent visit, I stopped the daytime formula and continued the nighttime formula for additional two weeks. She recovered after these two weeks.

参考文献

《黄帝内经》

REFERENCES

Huang Di Nei Jing

www.ingramcontent.com/pod-product-compliance
Lightning Source LLC
Chambersburg PA
CBHW041705210326
41598CB00007B/540

* 9 7 8 0 9 9 1 4 5 5 6 2 1 *